the
DIETER'S
PRAYER
book

SPIRITUAL POWER AND DAILY ENCOURAGEMENT

the
DIETER'S
PRAYER
book

HEATHER HARPHAM KOPP

WATERBROOK
PRESS

THE DIETER'S PRAYER BOOK
PUBLISHED BY WATERBROOK PRESS
2375 Telstar Drive, Suite 160
Colorado Springs, Colorado 80920
A division of Random House, Inc.

ISBN 1-57856-396-8

Copyright © 2000 by Heather Harpham Kopp

Published in association with the literary agency of Ann Spangler and Associates;
6260 Viewpoint Drive NE; Belmont, MI 49306.

Library of Congress Cataloging-in-Publication Data
Kopp, Heather Harpham, 1964-
    The dieter's prayer book : spiritual power and daily encouragement / Heather Harpham
Kopp.—1st ed.
        p. cm.
    Includes index.
    ISBN 1-57856-396-8 (hardback)
        1. Dieters—Prayer-books and devotions—English. I. Title.

BV4596.D53 K67 2000

242—dc21

                                                    00-061445

Printed in the United States of America
2001

10 9 8 7 6 5 4 3

Contents

Tending Our Bodies, Nourishing Our Souls

Recently Oprah Winfrey featured legendary soul diva Aretha Franklin on her show. During the course of the hour, Franklin discussed myriad personal and professional challenges, including her numerous divorces and her struggles with parenting. But the most telling—and in some ways most ordinary—revelation came when Oprah asked her, "So what would you say is the hardest thing you've ever faced?"

Franklin's quick answer: "Controlling my weight."

Of course Oprah nodded in perfect understanding as undoubtedly did millions of viewers, underscoring yet again that the battle for weight control knows no boundaries. Black or white, rich or poor, famous or ordinary, being defeated by food—outmaneuvered by our appetite and publicly humbled by our body shape—is a universal problem.

Solutions have been put forth since ancient times. Around 400 B.C., Hippocrates advised that "obese people and those desiring to lose weight" should eat their meals while they were still huffing and puffing from exercise. "They should, moreover, eat only once a day and take no baths and sleep on a hard bed and walk naked as long as possible."

Socrates' weight-control plan was more fun: dancing till dawn.

Today's solutions are more complicated—and expensive. In the past ten years the amount of money Americans have spent on diet programs and diet products has doubled to $30 billion. Diet books have never been more popular, with current titles touting a low-carb, high-protein regimen at the top of the *New York Times* bestseller lists. Add to that the scores of weight-loss options such as medication, nutritional coaching, psychotherapy, surgery, liposuction, and herbal remedies. It turns out there are as many ways to lose pounds as there are to gain them.

So how's it working for us?

Maybe we should all start dancing till dawn.

Recent studies show that Americans have never weighed more. The World Health Organization has announced that obesity is now a global epidemic. One in five adults is overweight enough to be considered clinically obese. Many cultures are obsessed with food and thinness—and yet many "weight-conscious" people grow fatter and more sedentary every year.

So are the diets failing us—or are we failing the diets?

The answer, of course, is neither and both. But before we go deeper, let me explain how I came to join the chorus of millions of people who are asking this question.

Meet the Real Cookie Monster

Once upon a time, I was one of those really skinny people, the kind who bug me now. I loved noodles and Cheetos and pizza with extra cheese. I ate what I wanted when I wanted. Or I forgot to eat. Even after giving birth twice in my early twenties, I still wore a size two. I couldn't understand why many of my friends had such a problem with weight gain. While they spent precious time and money trying to control their tendency to balloon, I thanked my metabolism, blessed my lucky genes, and ate Big Macs with abandon.

Then in my late twenties something began to change. At first, it was so gradual I shrugged it off. But it didn't end there. Year by year the arrow on my scale inched upward. My thighs widened. And my bottom—well, let's just say it took on a whole new texture and shape. I went from a size two to a size four. Then to a six. An eight. A ten. Then the size tens got tight…

2

You've probably heard about people who have been overweight so long that even after they lose some weight they can't see themselves as thin. I had the opposite problem. I was so used to being thin it took me years to actually realize I wasn't "the tiny one" anymore. Seemingly out of nowhere I'd turned into a person who could "stand to lose a few."

What happened next is predictable. I began to listen when the subject of dieting came up. I began to look at the fat and calorie counts on food packages. I began to really *look* in the mirror. And I started to resent naturally thin women who didn't struggle with this food thing and who flipped through racks of clothing looking for a size two or four.

Eventually I embarked on my own minivariation of the yo-yo dieting syndrome. While I never adhered religiously to one particular plan, I appropriated key principles and nutritional information into my eating routine. I cut back on carbohydrates and ate a lot of tuna. I gave up noodles and learned to tolerate celery. I lost several pounds.

But maintaining my new disciplines proved to be much harder than starting them. As long as I was being inspired by a book or a TV show, I did fine. But on the majority of days, when I reached down deep for the will power to make healthy choices, I came up empty. And boggled. How could a mushroom cheeseburger have so much power over me?

One day it dawned on me that food was not the problem and a new eating plan was not the answer. Every conscientious dieter stumbles on this fundamental realization sooner or later. We meet the real Cookie Monster…and she is us.

TURNING TOWARD THE LIGHT

Slowly I came to realize that I needed more than just information and determination to conquer my own weakness. I needed daily inspiration and help—and a power greater than my own inadequate will.

I had been writing books that led readers through Bible-based prayers—for marriage, for children, and even for the world's current influencers. By now there was no question in my mind that God's words were more powerful than my own. And when I prayed according to those words, incorporating the promises and principles of Scripture into my prayer life, something important and transforming took place.

One day it finally occurred to me that I should apply this same spiritual tool to my eating and health issues. If praying could help me in so many other "more important" areas of life, maybe it could actually help me when it came to weight control and pursuing a healthier lifestyle. The more I explored the dynamics of dieting and the role of my spirit, the more I realized that it was here—on the spiritual level—where the battle really lay.

The truth of the matter is that most of us know the dieting answers. We've read the books on what to eat and what not to eat, on the medical and nutritional whys. But it's the day-to-day behavior, attitude, and motivation challenges that do us in. In other words, it's not the broccoli we didn't eat or even the cookie-dough ice cream we did eat that swept our latest dieting resolution into the trash. It's those secret, tough-to-articulate, and absolutely lethal wars that rage in our heart.

Three thousand years ago Solomon, the sage of Israel, wrote, "Guard your heart, for it is the wellspring of life" (Prov. 4:23). Not your refrigerator. Not your fat-gram counter. Not your workout bag.

Your heart.

That's why this book starts there—at the wellspring of the heart. Any dieting book that is not about both body and soul is ultimately going to fail us, leave us impoverished and…well, hungry. Ultimately, I believe the struggle to gain control of our eating habits and to accept our own body involves a spiritual transformation.

For those of us who live in cultures of plenty, convenience, and excess, eating can become a substitute for soul tending. Many of use food to comfort ourselves, to fill our emptiness, to relieve boredom, or even to suppress anger. Our stomach gets fed, but our deeper soul hunger is not satisfied in the process. Perhaps this is why virtually every spiritual tradition includes fasting as a way to enhance spiritual awareness.

Food is not bad for us. In fact, our Creator meant for it to nourish and sustain us. But as with any other substance on earth, psychologically and physically food can also be abused. The addictive and impulse-driven person sees an unmet need and applies the most readily available medication. In many cases, this is food.

In the case of alcohol or drugs, abstinence may be the bottom-line solution. But because none of us can stop eating altogether, the struggle to master our eating habits is ongoing—and always at risk of being derailed. Making things more complicated is the fact that many people with weight problems suffer from depression, anxiety, and low self-esteem. And one of the easiest ways to cope with these feelings is to smother them by eating even more!

"Perhaps each of us has a starved place," writes Sue Bender in *Everyday Sacred.* "And each of us knows deep down what we need to fill that place. To find the courage to trust and honor the search, to follow the voice that tells us what we need to do, even when it doesn't seem to make sense, is a worthy pursuit."

That empty place inside could be called our "God tummy." And it is God's voice we must follow if we want to fill it. We may try to stuff a lot of things into that empty space—food, money, sex. But the only thing that truly satisfies is intimacy with God. Everything else leaves us hungry.

It's no coincidence that when Jesus was on earth, He declared several times, "I am the bread of life." And it was not merely for literary flair when God pleaded with people through the prophet Isaiah: "Why spend money on what is not bread, and your labor on what does not satisfy? Listen, listen to me, and eat what is good, and your soul will delight in the richest of fare" (Isa. 55:2).

With every hunger pang that has little to do with our stomach, God is calling us homeward, reminding us that He alone satisfies. And until we can be with Him in body and soul, we continue "feeding on Him in our hearts by faith," as the *Book of Common Prayer* puts it. As we do this, the same empty longing that makes us want to overeat will, if we let it, become a spiritual opportunity.

Are you willing to give God your full record of ups and downs, your driving and self-destructive desires and patterns, and ask Him to give you the hidden blessing that He sees there? If so, then you are ready for the kind of breakthroughs in your physical and spiritual life that this book is all about.

THE LANGUAGE OF CHANGE

"To pray is to change," writes Richard Foster in *Celebration of Discipline.* "Prayer is the central avenue God uses to transform us."

Once we break through the information overload and the girlfriend network buzz long enough, the role of our innermost being in our eating and self-care behavior becomes immediately apparent. *Of course that's how I work!* we realize. Every life-changing commitment starts there—in that "room of the heart" where spirit, will, emotions, and self-understanding meet to converse.

And prayer is the most natural language in that room. We pray about our fears. We pray about our hopes. We pray, perhaps, about major life decisions, such as who we will marry, what education or career we will pursue. We pray for those we love. Why, then, do so few of us pray about our dieting and health commitments?

Perhaps we think that these issues are too superficial, too vanity driven to merit a consciously tended conversation with our Creator. Does God really care if we gained ten pounds over the holidays? Are such personal physical concerns really occasions for prayer?

Yes! God clearly and repeatedly tells us to ask Him for what we need. In fact, He invites us to approach Him with the trust and humility of a child. "You do not have, because you do not ask God," Scripture says (James 4:2). When we call on God to help us with our eating, we are not trivializing God's role in our daily life, but enlarging it. Prayer is a sacred conversation with our Creator, an opportunity to listen for truth.

In Scripture we find clear, time-tested principles about food and hunger and our attitudes and behaviors concerning both. That's why these life-giving truths are the basis for the readings and prayers you'll find here. I hope you will use them to feed your spirit and nurture your inner life. However, I would also like to add a few words of caution:

First, it's important to take great care when applying spiritual principles to dieting. The last thing we need is more guilt! The readings in this book are not designed to shame you. (It's bad enough that I blew it and ate an entire bag of potato chips yesterday without having to call it a "sin against God.") Julian of Norwich wrote, "Our courteous Lord does not want his servants to despair even if they fall frequently and grievously. Our failing does not stop his loving us."

Second, these prayers are also not intended to focus so much on food that it is even further elevated in our mind. We already live in a food-obsessed culture. The food industry generates enough food for every man, woman, and child in the U.S. to consume 3,700 calories a day, and it spends $36 billion a year in advertising to try to convince us to eat it. The average child watches up to 10,000 food commercials a year—most of them for sugary, fatty, or salty foods! Our spiritual lives should not revolve around food. However, our struggle to eat healthily and take good care of ourselves can and should deeply involve our spiritual life.

Third, the trim body of our dreams is not a spiritual objective. Did you know the average American woman is five feet four inches, 144 pounds, and a size twelve? A far cry from the five-foot-eight-inch, 110-pound, size-two models glorified in glossy magazines. In fact, as you incorporate prayer disciplines into your daily life, you may find that a more complete and balanced view of God's design and purposes for you clearly indicate a body that will never grace a magazine cover—but is still a gift of beauty and grace to you and others.

Fourth, spiritual motivation should not replace medical information or nutritional advice. Recent books like David Meinz's *Eating by the Book,* Gwen Shamblin's *The Weigh Down Diet,* or Karen Kingsbury's *The Prism Weight-Loss Program* have done dieters the favor of applying biblical principles to weight control—along with providing medical information and nutritional guidelines. This book is not meant as a replacement for these or any other programs but as a spiritual tool to use with whatever weight-control approach works for you.

A Prayer a Day...

Deep down, every veteran dieter knows that diet books and programs have limited value because they don't permanently change our minds and hearts—which control our mouths, which lead to our stomachs. The promise of this book is that through prayer and the daily readings, and with God's help, you will gain spiritual power every day to do what you can't do on will power alone—make wise, healthy choices that will result in weight loss and better self-care.

This won't happen because you are reading the right book or because you're good at chanting the daily "Food for Thought" meditation. It will happen because you are encountering, inviting, and harnessing a power greater than your own—great enough to actually change you at your core. It will happen because you are calling upon a loving, powerful God!

But that's not all. I predict that you will also find yourself increasingly drawn to God in conversation and to the beautiful person—inside and out—that He is inviting you to become. Think about it. What God promises us through prayer can't be matched by any diet program:

Power. To deliver you from temptation. To raise in you a desire to live on a more spiritual level, full and content.

Relationship. You are not alone—especially when you face your toughest personal battles. God is your closest friend and ally. And guilt is the dieter's greatest enemy. Basking in the flow of God's continual river of unconditional love and acceptance is key to a healthy approach to dieting that outlasts any popular plan or program.

Affirming Words. God has something to say to you. He is knocking on your door! As you meditate on the wisdom of Scripture, you will hear the Spirit of God whispering in your ear all day long.

Guidance. As we pray, especially as we pray according to God's will, we learn. He is our great counselor and teacher. And we learn not just about how to lose weight, but how to live well, love well, and make every moment of our lives count.

The Big Picture. One of the most diminishing aspects of any diet regimen is that we risk becoming overly self-focused, body-obsessed, pound-conscious. We can lose sight of what really matters. Prayer gives us the perspective we need to see life in the light of eternity.

The old adage is still true: There's power in prayer. But here's a new adage you can begin to practice right now: A prayer a day keeps the weight away! More important, it brings you close to God's heart, where true solutions and endless love await.

PRAYERS

1 | Is "Diet" a Dirty Word?

Some trust in chariots and some in horses, but we trust in the name of the
LORD our God.

PSALM 20:7

You might read the verse above: Some trust in diets, some trust in calorie counting, but I trust in God's plans.

Many experts say that diets empower food, not people, because they're based on deprivation. And when we deprive ourselves of food we want, desperation takes over in time. We blow it. This is why the majority of books on weight control spend the first chapter declaring, "This is not a diet book!" (even if they use the word diet in the title).

To those who have failed with diets repeatedly, Gwen Shamblin writes in *The Weigh Down Diet,* "God has never asked anyone to eat food off a list, to count fat exchanges, or to take an appetite suppressant. You have just been applying the wrong medicine to this condition."

This isn't to say that all diets or weight-loss programs are bad. God can and *does* work in conjunction with these. What matters is that He is central to our plan. For the purpose of this book, let's redefine the word "diet" to mean:

- a **D**ecision to change the way I eat and the way I approach food
- an **I**nvitation to experience God's power and guidance
- an **E**ducated plan for long-term health and happiness
- a **T**rust that God will never give up on me or love me less—no matter what.

Food for Thought
"Diet" doesn't have to mean deprivation.

A Prayer for Power

Dear God,
I admit that I have come to both love
and hate the word "diet."
On the one hand, it represents hope for change.
On the other hand, it's like a sign flashing "Failure ahead!"
I don't want to simply embark on another faulty plan, Lord.
I want to embark on a journey with You
that is led by You and depends on Your power.
I can do nothing on my own!
And I don't want to just punish and deprive myself.
You and I both know where that leads: to rebellion and failure.
Show me the right path that will enable me to change.
Show me, as only You, who know me so intimately, can,
what works for me, what is healthy for me.
I want to think of this venture in positive terms, Lord—
not that I am signing up to be miserable or in want.
I want to learn to redirect my thinking, to feed my body
what it truly needs *when* it truly needs it.
And to feed my soul with the Bread of Life—You!
Today I place my future, my failures, my setbacks,
all of my hopes and plans into Your hands.
There alone will I find meaning
and true success in my life.
Amen.

2 | New Beginnings

Forget the former things; do not dwell on the past. See, I am doing a new thing!

ISAIAH 43:18-19

You are beginning a new journey of spirit and body. Larger spirit and smaller body, you hope! What a remarkable moment it is right now…you are reading in trust, waiting in expectation, listening…

New beginnings take so much courage, mostly because we remember all those other times we began again…and all the slips and fits and failures that happened next. How humbling to start over. Beginnings always call for bravery, because a beginning is a creative act. You want something to come into being that doesn't exist yet. Something new. Something better.

Here is a grace note for your first day of beginning again: God does it too, all the time! Every day is a new start. Every season, every year, every miracle of conception in a woman's womb… God reaches into the mysterious workings of earth almost as if to say, "I don't mind—I'll start again!"

The German poet Goethe once advised: "Whatever you can do or think you can, begin it. Boldness has genius, power, and magic in it."

The very fact that you are beginning again is a validation of God's presence and handiwork in your life. He has invited you to this page. He knows you and loves you, and at this moment He is ready to begin again to create His own beauty in your life.

Food for Thought
I can begin again!

A Prayer for Power

Dear God,
thank You that You are a God of new beginnings!
You didn't stop creating on the sixth day
but continue to create and recreate this world
and this person that I am.
I confess that it is hard for me to begin again.
I'm afraid to try to change
because I've failed so many times before.
But this I know: You don't waste any pain or any failure.
And You never give up!
You never throw up Your hands, walk away, and say,
"That's it! You'll never change!"
Instead, You are wholly and happily ready
every day to begin all over again with me.
Just as the sun rises new each day,
so do my opportunities for new beginnings and totally fresh starts.
Help me to remember that as I take small steps toward You,
You are always reaching out to help me
and You are rejoicing in my *progress.*
Your focus is not on the distance gained or the final destination.
Let's begin again, God.
Right now.
Amen.

3 | You Are What You Pray

Now faith is being sure of what we hope for and certain of what we do not see.

HEBREWS 11:1

There's some truth to the old saying "you are what you eat." But you are also what you pray.

Any change on the outside begins on the inside. "As he thinketh in his heart, so is he" (Prov. 23:7, KJV). Because the spirit and physical body are inseparably linked, the role of prayer in transformation can't be over-emphasized.

And neither can the role of faith. The apostle James tells us that if we doubt when we pray, we are like a ship tossed about on the sea. And how easy it is to doubt or become frustrated when you've been trying extra hard to eat right and exercise but aren't seeing the results you hoped for.

Today and every day God is calling you to a life of faith—and to commitment to prayers that ring with certainty. No matter what *you* see happening, God is at work. "So do not throw away your confidence," wrote the author of Hebrews, "it will be richly rewarded. You need to persevere so that when you have done the will of God, you will receive what he has promised" (Heb. 10:35-36).

Food for Thought

You are what you what eat, what you think, what you say, what you do,
and what you pray.

A PRAYER FOR POWER

Dear God,
today I come to You in faith,
asking for what I fear I may lack—
great faith!
Help me, Lord, to understand
how I can stand firmly on shaky ground,
believe in what I can't see,
trust in what I can only hope for.
Bathe me in Your faithful love
that I might in turn love You more faithfully.
I surrender myself and my body to You right now,
along with all my expectations.
In exchange, may I receive from You
a confidence that can't be shaken.
Make me a woman of faith, Lord.
I am not strong enough to create all my own success,
but I believe that You will accomplish
all the good plans You have for me.
Amen.

4 | Five Pounds by Sunday

It is not good to have zeal without knowledge, nor to be hasty and miss the way.

PROVERBS 19:2

So. Your best friend's wedding, which you so wanted to look marvelous for, is just around the corner, but those unsightly five pounds you hoped to lose by then are still around your middle.

It's tempting to panic at times like these, to have "zeal without knowledge"—as did the woman who prepared for a cruise by wrapping herself in cellophane and then jogging ten miles. She ended up in the hospital and missed the vacation.

When you're feeling impatient with your weight-loss progress, don't panic and lose your head. Real change takes time, and shortcuts will likely lead you to "miss the way" altogether.

When it comes to changing your eating and exercise habits, slow and steady is best. Most experts recommend that you lose no more than one to two pounds a week and consider a half-pound a week great progress.

It helps to remember that your goal is bigger than inches or pounds can measure—and it's more important than any special occasion. Your goal is to become all that God created you to be—and to develop a patient spirit as part of the beautiful person you are.

Food for Thought
The fast track to lasting change is the slow one.

A Prayer for Power

Dear God,
thank You that even when I am impatient or foolish,
when I am so zealous to see results
that I rush things and miss the way altogether,
You forgive me and help me
to find the right path again.
Today I pray that You would grant me
the wisdom, will, and patience
to persevere in the process of change.
Help me to accept where I am right now.
With Your power at work within me,
I can keep my eyes on my true goal:
to become the best me I can be—for You!
Today I embrace Your loving intentions for me,
and I put all my hope in Your good and perfect timing.
Amen.

5 | When God Looks at You

How beautiful you are, my darling! Oh, how beautiful!...like a lily among thorns.

SONG OF SONGS 1:15; 2:2

What do you think God sees when He looks at you?

Though some days you feel like a walking ruin, your loving God sees the real you—a work of art, a lily among thorns.

If you find those words hard to take in, you're not alone. For many of us, the choice to accept approval and honest admiration requires enormous courage, especially if we usually spend our energy focusing on our shortcomings. Frances de Sales advised, "Be patient with everyone, but above all with yourself; do not be disheartened by your imperfections, but always rise up with fresh courage."

Today ask God for the courage to simply receive His loving gaze upon you without turning away or refusing His affections. He knows you completely, so there's no need to hide. And His heart toward you is passionate, constant, and tender. Hear His whisper in your ear all day long:

"Oh, how beautiful you are!"

Food for Thought
The One who knows me absolutely
thinks I am absolutely beautiful.

A Prayer for Power

Dear God,
thank You that You see all the way through
to my very core
and You love every part of me.
Even when I am weak, selfish,
or unattractive in spirit,
You still call me Your beauty and beloved!
Because I know
I am already lovely in Your sight,
I can "work" on becoming even more so
with confidence and joy.
Because You have called me beautiful,
grant me the power and the courage today
to believe it
and to touch every person I meet
with grace and hope.
Amen.

6 | Thin for Thin's Sake?

All a man's ways seem innocent to him, but motives are weighed by the LORD.

PROVERBS 16:2

Paige, a member of Overeaters Anonymous, told a reporter for *Life* magazine, "I used to make up these diets for myself and lose weight real fast, and people would say, 'You'll get real sick if you don't stop eating that way,' and I can remember consciously thinking, 'As long as I'm thin in the casket and people walk by and say, "Oh, my gosh, look how thin she is," I really wouldn't mind dying on a diet.'"

An extreme story, but did you find yourself relating?

Health experts (and God!) agree: To achieve lasting change in the dieting department our primary motivation must be to become more healthy—not just thin. If our reason for changing is that we're terrified of being fat, our efforts will ultimately fail or may even spiral into an eating disorder.

As Elyse Fitzpatrick points out in *Love to Eat, Hate to Eat,* "While there are some biblical concerns that can be brought to bear on our health and eating habits—such as…thinking about your life in the way that He does, and learning to discern whether your eating habits are godly—the whole matter of thinness for thinness' sake isn't one of them."

God's not opposed to your being trim. But He doesn't want you to sacrifice your health on the altar of thinness. God's goal for you is the best of everything—right motives, healthy choices, and a body you enjoy.

Food for Thought
Thinness for the sake of thinness is a thin motive.

A Prayer for Power

Dear God,
if there's one area where I need Your power
it is in this area of right motivation!
I confess that more often than not
I have mixed motives in my dieting quest.
I want to be healthy, yes,
but I also want to be thin because thin is "better."
You know I'm incapable of always having right motives.
But You, Lord, are able to purify me!
Guide me, remind me, redirect me, reveal the truth to me.
I offer You my heart, with all its tricky devices,
and I ask You to cleanse it by the power of Your Holy Spirit.
May I pursue right motives because they matter to me,
and because they matter to You.
Giver of wisdom and insight,
Giver of every good gift,
grant me wisdom and motives that come from a pure heart
that I might glorify You in every way.
Amen.

7 | The Trouble with Denial

You, O LORD, keep my lamp burning; my God turns my darkness into light.

PSALM 18:28

One of the most seductive forces at work in the life of an overeater is denial. Denial is a lie we tell ourselves, an invisible (at least to ourselves) barrier of protection that says, "Not here, not now, not me—no way!" If we can keep ourselves in the dark about how much we really eat or how unhealthy we really are, for example, we don't have to face the challenge of fixing it.

Meanwhile, the problem gets worse with neglect. "You cannot afford the luxury of defensiveness, and you cannot afford the luxury of lies and denial," writes Phillip McGraw in *Life Strategies*. "Denial, after all, is what kills dreams. It kills hope. It kills what might have a real chance to overcome a problem had the solution just been pursued in time."

Usually we're in denial about what's keeping us in a pattern of failure. Dietra, a victim of sexual abuse as a child, had been obese for twelve years before she finally admitted that she used her weight to keep men away, to feel safe. As she faced this truth, she was able to see a clearer path toward a healthier life.

Ask God if there is any corner of your heart that you keep hidden in the shadows of denial. Try this: Look yourself in the mirror and say what you least want to hear. Start your declaration like this: "Because I am my Lord's beloved child, I have the strength to say truthfully what I least want to admit about myself, and that is…"

As you honestly face the truth and nothing but the truth, God can begin to turn your pain into hope, your darkness into light.

Food for Thought
Is denial denying me success and health?

A Prayer for Power

Dear God,
why is it so hard to face myself?
I imagine that I'm being honest,
only to realize that I'm hiding
a large corner of my heart from my own eyes.
Foolishly I imagine that I'm hiding it from Yours as well.
But, of course, You see everything.
You know everything about me.
"You perceive my thoughts from afar....
Before a word is on my tongue
you know it completely" (Ps. 139:2,4).
Right now, Lord, I'm ready to look
at whatever truth You want to reveal to me.
I know that when I choose to lie to myself,
I deny You the chance to heal me and help me.
Thank You that You only want to help!
Thank You that whatever painful reality I must face,
You will face it with me.
You understand.
You care.
You're here.
Amen.

8 | Destined for Fatness?

My frame was not hidden from you when I was made in the secret place.

PSALM 139:15

One of the greatest debates in the dieting world is whether or not some people are genetically destined to be fat. Their mother was fat, and their grandmother Lois before her.

Science supports the idea that much about you—from the rate at which you metabolize food, to the "fat spots" where excess weight rests, to the size of your skeletal frame—is indeed inherited. These factors play a part in how you lose weight and at what rate and where. You may be genetically predisposed to be heavier than your size-four friend. However, the question of whether or not there is a "fat" gene is still up for grabs.

Researchers at New York City's Rockefeller University announced in 1999 that they had discovered a genetic mutation in obese mice that essentially keeps a mutant mouse's brain from knowing its stomach is full. Although the discovery was greeted with enthusiasm, it's a long way from mice to men, and it will take years to develop any practical application to you and me.

While some overweight people find comfort in such theories as a fat gene, the idea leaves many others feeling defeated, hopeless. *Why try then?*

But there are at least three encouraging truths that hold true: God didn't make any mistakes when He created you. The basics principles of weight gain and loss remain the same: 3,500 calories equal a pound! And finally, God knows exactly how you're made, and He's committed to helping you become all He has in mind.

Food for Thought
Genes play a role, but God plays the lead.

A Prayer for Power

Dear God,
as You know, some days I wish
I looked different than I do,
and I wonder if something got mixed up
when You were choosing traits from my parents
to give to me.
How good it is to be reminded, Lord,
that You knew exactly what You were doing
and that You had me—exactly *this* me—
in mind long before I came to exist!
So today I present myself to You—
all that I am, genetically and physically—
with a grateful heart.
Help me to be a good steward of my body.
Because You designed it,
I want to celebrate, nurture, and respect it.
By Your power at work in me,
I praise You for every molecule, gene, and freckle!
Amen.

9 | Go to the Source

He will be the sure foundation for your times, a rich store of salvation and wisdom and knowledge; the fear of the LORD is the key to this treasure.

ISAIAH 33:6

Everyone seems to have a different plan for weight-loss success: Go off carbohydrates, cut out all sugar, weigh yourself every day, don't weigh yourself every day, take care of your inner child, get in touch with the skinny person buried deep inside…

How can you sort through the cacophony of advice? It might sound simplistic, but the best place to start is with the greatest fitness "guru" ever—and His best-selling book. Believe it or not, the Bible is a "rich store of wisdom" for learning how to live well. And the surest foundation for any healthful venture is an intimate relationship with the One who created you. After all, He alone has complete and intimate knowledge about how your particular, unique body works.

In *The Weigh Down Diet,* Gwen Shamblin puts it this way: "God is the genius of behavior modification. He programs us to long for this correct weight…and he does not reward Band-Aid approaches."

God's Word addresses all kinds of issues, from how to avoid self-indulgence and gluttony to how to develop true inner beauty. So next time you're sorting through advice from the experts, don't forget to go to the ultimate Source. By His Spirit of truth, God can lead you to discover and develop what works best for you.

Food for Thought
God is the only diet "guru" with the inside scoop on you.

A Prayer for Power

Dear God,
I know that, first of all,
You are the sure foundation
of healthy, fulfilling, and meaningful living!
Grant me a willing spirit
to make the most of what You reveal to me,
and help me to apply sound principles
in caring for my mind and my body.
I never want to waste my time on silly ploys or bad advice.
Instead, I will listen for Your voice,
and I will hold up every idea to the light of Your Word.
Thank You that You are my closest confidant
and my favorite partner.
You are always on my side,
and You are always right!
Stay close to me today, and bless me with the treasures of
Your presence,
Your comfort,
Your wisdom,
Your power.
Amen.

10 | More Than Conquerors

No, in all these things we are more than conquerors through him who loved us.

ROMANS 8:37

Do you feel like a conqueror today?

You are! Even if you feel defeated and victory seems far away. If there's one truth you cling to in the coming months, let it be this: Nothing—no amount of fat or failure!—can separate you from God's love or rob you of the conquering power you inherited from Him.

Listen to what William Law writes in *An Appeal to All That Doubt:*

> Here is opened to us the true reason of the whole process of our Saviour's incarnation, passion, death, resurrection, and ascension into Heaven. It was because fallen man was to go through all these stages as necessary parts of his return to God; and therefore, if man was to go out of his fallen state there must be a son of this fallen man, who, as a head and fountain of the whole race, could do all this—could go back through all these gates and so make it possible for all the individuals of human nature, as being born of Him, to inherit His conquering nature and follow Him through all these passages to eternal life.

Because of Christ's work on the cross, *you have inherited His conquering nature.* Use it! Live in His love, walk in His wake, and victory will be yours.

Food for Thought
Through Christ's power in me, I can conquer any problem!

A Prayer for Power

Dear God,
help me to always remember and lay hold of
the victory that can be—that is!—mine in Christ Jesus.
Too often I live like someone defeated,
someone who is powerless to change.
Like a soldier who forgets his sword,
I neglect your Word, leave Your love at the door.
It doesn't have to be that way—and it won't be anymore!
For I am convinced
—yes, absolutely and irrevocably convinced!—
that neither death nor life,
(not cancer, accidents, difficult relationships, or disappointments)
neither angels nor demons,
(not cults, spiritual oppression, or evil in the media)
neither the present nor the future,
(not any crisis looming now or any tragedy yet to come)
nor any powers,
(not political, financial, military, cultural, or even culinary!)
neither height nor depth,
(not great success or crushing defeat)
nor anything else in all creation,
will be able to separate me from the love of God
that is in Christ Jesus my Lord (from Rom. 8:38-39).
Amen!

31

11 | Temple Tending

*Or don't you know that your body is the temple of the Holy Spirit, who lives in
you and was given to you by God? You do not belong to yourself, for God bought
you with a high price. So you must honor God with your body.*

1 CORINTHIANS 6:19-20, NLT

Usually we think of this scripture as it applies to sexuality. But it means so
much more than that. If we really consider our bodies to be the home of
the Holy Spirit, the place where He "hangs out" all the time, then we have
to take seriously how well we are keeping up that home. Would you want
to live in a house where there was no discipline, where the grass out front
was overgrown, the TV blared constantly, the paint was old and peeling,
the unwashed dishes covered every counter?

Sheri Rose Shepherd writes in *7 Ways to Build a Better You,* "How do
we honor God with our body if we trash His temple?... If we're exhausted
all the time or sick all the time, how do we have the energy to serve Him?
If He has called us to be of sound mind, to have a good attitude, and to
be used by Him, we obviously have to be healthy in order to do that."

It's easy, isn't it, to forget whom we belong to, whose temple we are
tending? Today let the truth of who dwells within you be the motive for
making healthy choices. As you honor God with your body, He will
delight to honor you with the conscious presence and power of His precious Holy Spirit.

Food for Thought
Is the Holy Spirit at home in your body?

A Prayer for Power

Dear God,
welcome to my heart,
Your home!
How honored I am to know
that Your Holy Spirit lives in me!
May this knowledge constantly remind and inspire me
to treat my physical body with reverence—
not to worship it, but to worship You
and Your indwelling presence.
My body is just temporary, Lord.
Someday You will give me a new body,
and I will see You face to face.
I can't wait!
In the meantime, I offer my thoughts, my actions,
my words, and my attitudes—
all of me—to You.
Make me a living sacrifice,
a lovely testament to the power to be found
only in You.
Amen.

12 | The Strength of My Heart

*My flesh and my heart may fail, but God is the strength of my heart
and my portion forever.*

PSALM 73:26

Are you tired today? Exhausted from too many days on the front lines?

Whenever we try to improve ourselves, there is a constant temptation to strive toward our goals in our own strength. Our "flesh and…heart" fail, and we end up exhausted and disillusioned.

It's a paradox, isn't it? On one hand, we must take responsibility for our choices, run the race well, and beat our bodies into submission (1 Cor. 9:24-27). Yet we can do nothing apart from God's power. He wants us to be completely dependent on Him!

Hannah Whitall Smith wrote in *The Christian's Secret of a Happy Life*, "Be generous in your self-surrender!… Be glad and eager to throw yourself headlong into His dear arms, and to hand over the reins of government to Him. Whatever there is of you, let Him have it all."

As you go about your day today, look for places, ways, and times to abandon yourself to God and make Him "the strength of your heart." Even as you do your part by obeying Him, throw yourself "headlong into His dear arms," and you'll begin to experience the kind of surrender that yields true victory.

Food for Thought
Let His strength be the strength of your heart.

A Prayer for Power

Dear Lord,
help me to understand this glorious truth:
Although I am called to exert effort on Your behalf,
and mine,
I am also called to depend completely
upon You and Your strength.
Make Your strength my strength today.
You know how weak I am,
how quickly my energy flags
when my arms are not linked with Yours,
when my soul is running on empty.
Fill me with Your Holy Spirit,
with Your miraculous power and strength.
I surrender all that I am—
and all that I am not, as well—
to You, Lord.
Take me as I am.
Make me wholly Yours,
and I will be whole.
Amen.

13 | Free Indeed

It is for freedom that Christ has set us free. Stand firm, then, and do not let yourselves be burdened again by a yoke of slavery.

GALATIANS 5:1

We all need to be rescued sometimes, but the best emancipations in life come when we are rescued from a brutal and destructive slave master who lives inside us. Isn't it comforting to know that God sent His Son to earth to win for us just that kind of freedom! "So if the Son sets you free, you will be free indeed" (John 8:36).

The fact is, we were created for freedom, not slavery. And prayer is one way we can tap into God's emancipation power. By His Spirit, alive in our hearts, He is able to break down spiritual and emotional strongholds that we don't even see—like bitterness, self-loathing, stubbornness, negative thinking, and fear. With His help, we never have to slide back into bondage.

Find fresh motivation for your commitments today by recalling the personal liberations you've already experienced. What did you reach for? What did you leave behind? Then ponder God's promise of power to deliver you from future addictions and compulsions of every kind. Let a lifestyle of freedom take up residence in your heart, filling every corner. And when the old habits (masquerading as worthy pleasures) come knocking, stand firm in your liberty. Name those deceitful appeals for what they are: slave owners! Ugly and oppressive burdens! Miserable yokes of shame!

Remember who you are: freedom's child, free indeed!

Food for Thought
God chose to set me free; only I can choose not to be.

A Prayer for Power

Dear God,
today I claim Your promise
that You are able to free me from anything inside or outside myself
that may be holding me captive.
I know that You are stronger
than any habit, dependency, or destructive pull in my life.
When my enemies—
temptations and old, bothersome habits of all kinds—
attack, You are ready to save me if only I will call out for help.
Save me today, I pray.
Help me to do my part to stand firm and not slide back into slavery.
I don't want to live there anymore.
Awesome God, because You have called me to freedom,
I am free indeed!
Amen.

14 | A Giving Strategy

If you spend yourselves in behalf of the hungry and satisfy the needs of the oppressed, then your light will rise in the darkness, and your night will become like the noonday.

ISAIAH 58:10

Have you ever thought about giving as a dieting strategy? It makes sense, doesn't it? If you want to eat less, give away more food!

Mother Teresa wrote in *A Gift for God,* "The same way Jesus allows himself to be broken and given to us as food, we, too, must divide and share what we have with others."

It's so easy to get caught up in trying to "save" what is ours—our time, our resources, our energies. But our insecurities can quickly turn "saving" into hoarding or shortsighted obsessions.

Here's a heaven-sent giving strategy for today: As we turn our focus away from our own appetites and "spend ourselves" on behalf of the truly needy and oppressed, God acts on our behalf. The clamor of our personal needs recedes as we gain a new perspective. Petty preoccupations fall away. We make room for something better—like a miracle!

Make giving a regular part of your lifestyle by sponsoring a hungry child, volunteering at a food kitchen, or giving regularly to a local food bank. Ask God to show you a creative way to divide what you have and give out of your abundance. And see if your own stingy stomach doesn't feel a little less greedy!

Food for Thought
As I give from what I have, I will be rich with less.

A Prayer for Power

Dear God,
how much I need Your help
to turn my self-interest outward.
My problem is too much food,
but for so many that You love, the problem is just the opposite!
Forgive me, Lord, for my shortsightedness.
Right now I choose to spend my hunger on someone
who is truly lacking the essentials.
Thank You for the satisfaction and enlightenment
that You promise I will experience through generous giving.
And thank You that, through me,
You are ready and willing to bless my world
with comfort and abundance.
Amen.

15 | Pray for Me

Therefore confess your sins to each other and pray for each other so that you may be healed. The prayer of a righteous man is powerful and effective.

JAMES 5:16

As groups like Alcoholics Anonymous have discovered, people trying to overcome addictions or to change habits need at least three essential things: encouragement, accountability, and spiritual power. And God would add a fourth: prayer.

The apostle James tells us to pray for each other "so that you may be healed." And isn't healing what we're really after? Healing of compulsions, healing of old hurts, healing of our own self-indulgent spirit?

It's easy to keep prayer in our back pocket as a last resort—after we've put a lock on the fridge and asked our husband to hide the key; after we've yo-yoed up and down the scale for the fifth time. But God says that the prayer of a "righteous" person—read that "clothed in Christ"—is powerful and effective.

Find a friend of faith who will partner with you on your dieting journey. Hold each other accountable, and hold one another up in prayer to the God who has all power. Why not call each other once a day to pray briefly over the phone? Why not look for encouragement from Scripture to share? That kind of prayer friendship between righteous dieters is powerful and effective. God said so!

Food for Thought
Friends hold each other up—and let divine power in.

A Prayer for Power

Dear God,
first I want to thank You for being
my very best Friend.
When I am discouraged, You lift my head.
When I am lost, You lead the way.
When I am hurt by life or another person,
You listen to me talk into the night.
Thank You, God!
Because You are my friend,
You care about sending me friends
that I can see and touch and laugh with.
How much I need their help and companionship,
especially from those who struggle with
the same things I struggle with.
Continue to bless my life with such friends, God,
even as I continue to try to become
the best kind of friend I can possibly be.
Like a Matchmaker who loves His job,
match me up with hearts that will link with mine
in a common purpose.
Give us the wisdom and tenacity to hold each other accountable
and the grace to hold each other up in prayer to You.
Amen.

16 | More Power to Me!

I pray also that the eyes of your heart may be enlightened in order that you may know the hope to which he has called you, the riches of his glorious inheritance in the saints, and his incomparably great power for us who believe.

EPHESIANS 1:18-19

Power is a big deal these days. We go to power lunches. We wear power suits. Kids watch Power Rangers, and Christians watch the "Hour of Power."

But what is power, really? And how do we get it?

Power is a force of energy that can be brought to bear on something. The greatest possible power source on earth is God's Spirit. The apostle Paul called His power "incomparably great." That means it can't even be compared to something human or imagined.

God's power is not magic. It's better. It's miraculous! Paul goes on to tell the Ephesians, "That power is like the working of his mighty strength, which he exerted in Christ when he raised him from the dead" (Eph. 1:19-20).

Unlike worldly power, God's power is only holy and good. And here's the best part: He wants you to hunger for it and to wield it in every area of your life where you feel weak. "Be strong in the Lord and in his mighty power," Paul exhorted (Eph. 6:10).

Today ask God to clothe you in His power. Power to love. Power over your appetites and over sin. Power to be raised up to new life.

Food for Thought
It's time to get power hungry.

A Prayer for Power

Dear God,
I can't fathom the kind of power
You have at Your disposal.
And to think that through Your Son,
I have access to that power!
I want to use it, Lord.
I want to want it for all the right reasons.
You promised that if anyone
asked for Your Holy Spirit, You would give it.
So here I am, knocking, asking.
Give me Your Spirit, and fill me with power.
Yes, clothe me with power from on high.
Be powerful through me.
Be powerful in spite of me.
Be powerful in those moments when I am weakest.
Give me faith to believe in Your power
and the grace to seize every opportunity
to let it accomplish Your will for my life.
More power to me!
Amen.

17 | What's on God's Mind?

Give to Caesar what is Caesar's, and to God what is God's.

MATTHEW 22:21

Do you start every day asking God for strength and go to bed every night apologizing for blowing it? Do you feel you must repent to God every time you eat a brownie? Miss a workout?

It's possible to overspiritualize our quest for a healthy life. When the Pharisees asked if they should pay taxes, Jesus was blunt, saying in essence, "That's not a spiritual issue; it's a civic duty." In the same way, it's possible to give too much priority and ascribe too much spiritual significance to our dieting.

Granted, our journey *is* spiritual as well as physical, and we need God's grace and strength daily. However, our caloric intake shouldn't be the first thing that comes up every time we pray. And our eating successes or failures on any given day shouldn't shape our spiritual stance toward God.

In most cases our spiritual commitments in other areas of life should be far more important than our quest for a healthy body. Our relationships with people have eternal consequences, as does exercising our spiritual gifts.

Ask God today if there's any area of life that has been eclipsed by your eating concerns. Give your body the attention it's due, but also seek to discover what's on God's mind for you today and for the rest of your life.

Food for Thought
How can I align my focus with God's?

A Prayer for Power

Dear God,
today I offer my heart and mind to You.
I am open and ready, waiting to see
what is on Your mind for me.
Forgive me if I have focused on my body and eating
to the exclusion of more important things.
I know that You never turn me away when I seek Your help
and that what might seem trivial to some is important to You
if it's important to me.
Just as You care, Lord, about each care of mine,
I want to care about what's important to You.
Speak to me today as I go about my routines;
whisper Your truth into my spirit.
By Your power at work in my life,
may I find ways to create balance and harmony,
to attend to what matters right now
without neglecting what is important in light of eternity.
Only You know my whole life, Lord.
Only You know exactly what I need each day.
Show me the right paths.
Lead me gently, Shepherd of my heart,
and I will follow.
Amen.

18 | Honest Scales

Honest scales and balances are from the LORD; all the weights in the bag are of his making.

PROVERBS 16:11

When God's Word talks about "honest scales," he's not referring to modern bathroom scales (women in Bible times never weighed themselves—imagine!). And yet, the fact remains that He loves the truth and doesn't endorse scales that lie.

"All a man's ways seem right to him," Scripture says, "but the LORD weighs the heart. To do what is right and just is more acceptable to the LORD than sacrifice" (Prov. 21:2-3).

Is your favorite scale the one that weighs you a couple pounds lighter than you really are? Join the club! But who's fooling whom? And does it matter?

Many experts believe that women should do away with bathroom scales altogether. "We understand that it is odd to live in a weight obsessed world without occasionally stepping on a scale," writes Jane R. Hirschmann, author of *When Women Stop Hating Their Bodies*. "It is important to remember, however, that we never really used these scales to tell us how much we *weighed*. We used them to tell us if we were *good* or *bad*."

Next time you're busy worrying about your weight and making grand plans to get trim, remember that God is quietly weighing your heart. He's much more concerned with your integrity than with your sacrifice of food. No matter what the scale says, He's already decided that you are beloved in His sight—whether or not you feel you've been "good."

Food for Thought
Most of what really matters can't be measured in pounds.

A Prayer for Power

God, help me today to care as much
about my heart's "weight"
as I do about my body's weight.
Thank You that because Your scales never lie
and Your bottom line is always love,
I can stand before You with confidence
no matter how "good" or "bad" I've been lately.
Show me how to truthfully measure
the progress of both my soul
and my body.
For I know that the one
will someday pass away,
while the other will matter forever.
Amen.

19 | Fools Forgiven Here

I have sinned greatly in what I have done. Now, O LORD, I beg you, take away the guilt of your servant. I have done a very foolish thing.

2 SAMUEL 24:10

It's been said that the key to success is to be good at failing.

In the midst of our own mistakes, failures, and even foolish rebellion against our own goals, great opportunities to change our course often present themselves. And God is interested in one thing: full restoration. He doesn't forgive us more deeply if we first beat our heads against the wall, throw in the towel, or decide just to give up. Failure is part of the long path to success. It's our response to failure that makes all the difference.

When the apostle Peter failed, Jesus gently restored him, but not by saying, "I can't believe you did that!" and going over each incident when Peter denied Him. Instead, He affirmed what He knew to be good and true about Peter, nudging him to see for himself by his answer to Jesus' question, "Do you love me?"

Judas, on the other hand, who underestimated God's loving-kindness and forgiveness, punished himself pointlessly and irreversibly by taking his own life in guilt and shame.

When you waver, reach for Him. When you start sinking, call out His name. He'll be there, and He'll welcome you back into His arms just as readily as He did the first time you stumbled.

Food for Thought
When you fail, run *for* God, not *from* Him.

A Prayer for Power

Dear God,
today I am so thankful for Your Word,
which promises that "You are forgiving and good, O Lord,
abounding in love to all who call to you" (Ps. 86:5).
Forgive me for my failures,
grant me Your goodness,
let Your love abound to me, O Lord!
Help me never to run away from You
when I've failed or sinned,
but compel me always to run toward You, as Peter did,
and ask You gratefully and confidently for forgiveness.
No matter what I've done, or how badly I've blown it,
You promise that if I confess my sin to You,
You will be faithful and just and will forgive me
my sins and purify me from all unrighteousness (1 John 1:9).
Today, by Your power working in me,
I don't have to live with regret and fear.
Thank You, kind and compassionate Lord!
Amen.

20 | Is Fudge Sinful?

Don't you see that whatever enters the mouth goes into the stomach and then out of the body? But the things that come out of the mouth come from the heart, and these make a man "unclean."

MATTHEW 15:17-18

Jesus made it clear that no food in itself is sinful, but sin comes from inside our hearts. So does that mean it's not possible to sin with food?

No. The Bible gives us clear guidelines about when our eating might become sinful. The apostle Paul wrote, "'Everything is permissible for me'—but not everything is beneficial" (1 Cor. 6:12). In other words, I'm allowed to eat that brownie, but is it good for me? He went on to say, "'Everything is permissible for me'—but I will not be mastered by anything" (v. 12). If we feel we can't say no to a certain food, then it has too much power over us.

Paul also told the Romans, "If anyone regards something as unclean, then for him it is unclean" (Rom. 14:14). In other words, it might be okay for your friend Sally to eat cheesecake. But if you've decided that cheesecake is wrong for you, then you should be true to your conscience and not eat it.

Remember, God wants you to live in freedom! Use wisdom, and eat what is beneficial and "good for you." Ask God to reveal what is "sin" for you personally. He does not want you to be mastered by or controlled by anything other than His Holy Spirit. Then you can eat without worry or fear!

Food for Thought
Food isn't sinful; we are.

A Prayer for Power

Dear God,
I am so glad that no food is
sinful in and of itself.
I want to get to the point where I recognize
that food is not my enemy.
Bring me to health in my thinking in this area.
Help me not to overspiritualize my dieting
yet also to heed the gentle nudgings of Your Spirit.
Reveal to me where there is any sin
in my relationship with food or anything else.
I only want one master of my life—
and that's You.
Thank You that You care about *me*,
not the foods I eat.
You want me to be free, to live a life of self-control and joy.
By Your power at work within me,
I know that I can live each day with a clean conscience.
I want to be true to You and true to myself
in what I say, do, and eat today.
Give me Your grace and wisdom, Lord.
Amen.

21 | A Dangerous Business

You were taught...to be made new in the attitude of your minds; and to put on the new self, created to be like God in true righteousness and holiness.

In *Clinging: The Experience of Prayer*, Emilie Griffin writes, "Prayer is, after all, a very dangerous business. For all the benefits it offers of growing closer to God, it carries with it one great element of risk: the possibility of change."

We might ask, why would change be a risk? Isn't change what we're after? Maybe. Maybe not. The truth is that we have this strange tendency to seek change, all the while resisting it with every fiber of our being.

God tells us that the moment we receive Christ as Savior we become new creatures. But He also tells us to "put on the new self" and "be made new"—in short, to pursue a process of change.

Let's face it: Change is hard. It's so difficult, in fact, that we often avoid it even when it would improve our life dramatically. Millions of books are written to address our heartfelt desire: *I want to change—in my marriage, my job, my faith, my parenting, my eating—but I can't seem to make it happen!*

That, of course, is where God comes in. And that too is the danger—and the promise—of prayer: real change through the power of the Holy Spirit at work within us. This doesn't mean that if we pray, change will happen magically or without effort. But it does mean that we have good reason to pray in faith and to reach for change, confident that when we do, God's Spirit is reaching back to us.

Food for Thought
Pray, if you dare to change.

A Prayer for Power

Dear God,
how I praise You for the power of prayer.
It is dangerous, yes,
when I don't sincerely want to change.
But today I embrace it as a glorious risk
that I am willing and wanting to take.
As I spend time with You,
change me through and through.
Plant a desire for dramatic change deep inside my spirit.
I know that I cannot achieve lasting, true change apart from Your help,
apart from time spent in Your transforming presence.
Make me willing to do hard things, God.
I want to be faithful to cooperate
with every new and good thing You are trying to do in me.
I want to be unrecognizable to myself!
I want to be completely transformed,
to take up the beautiful calling of that new creature You made me
the day You saved me.
Amen.

22 | Pound Prejudice

If you show special attention to the man wearing fine clothes and say, "Here's a good seat for you," but say to the poor man, "You stand there" or "Sit on the floor by my feet," have you not discriminated among yourselves and become judges with evil thoughts?

JAMES 2:3-4

At some time or another, all of us have been guilty of discriminating against other people based on their clothing, social status, financial status—or weight. Often without meaning to, we buy into the myth that a thin person is somehow more valuable than one who is obese.

Sue, thirty-eight and once 100 pounds overweight, has felt this kind of discrimination firsthand. "People think because you're fat that it's okay to be rude." She remembers eating an ice cream cone and being accosted by a total stranger who said, "You certainly don't need that."

Carol, who at forty-nine has lost 116 pounds, declares: "Prejudice against overweight people is the last type of 'acceptable' discrimination."

Of course, pound prejudice isn't aimed only at the obese. Consider the heavy woman who avoids the size-four gal in her Bible study, assuming she's vain, arrogant, and shallow. Or how about the very overweight woman who mocks her friend's heartfelt desire to lose those stubborn ten pounds?

Ask yourself, What can I do today to not only accept someone who is different, but to love, include, and embrace her?

Food for Thought
God's love is the same size for everyone.

A Prayer for Power

I thank You, God,
that You do not discriminate among the people You have created,
no matter their religious background,
social status, gender, race, color—or size!
In You we are equal—
and equally loved.
Forgive me for those times when I have
unfairly judged another person because she or he
was different from me.
Because of the way You love me,
I know that there is great power
in unconditional love and acceptance.
Today, grant me Your power
so that I will love, reach out to, and encourage
every son or daughter of Yours
who comes across my path.
Amen.

23 | Self-Control

Like a city whose walls are broken down is a man who lacks self-control.

PROVERBS 25:28

When we lose control of ourselves, we're wide open to attack and to getting trampled by our enemies—like laziness and self-indulgence. God can give us strength, and His Holy Spirit gives us power. But *we* have to choose self-control.

In 1990 a New Jersey real-estate investor who tipped the scales at 298 pounds got fed up with his lack of self-control. His answer? He offered a $25,000 reward to the chosen charity of anyone who spotted him eating in a restaurant—his greatest weakness. At first it worked. He lost 114 pounds. Then he gained back 80. Today at 5'8" and 310 pounds, he no longer offers the reward but doesn't rule out doing so again someday.

The moral of the story: No amount of outside pressure can take the place of self-control.

Oswald Chambers wrote in *My Utmost for His Highest,* "The battle is lost or won in the secret places of the will before God, never first in the external world.... If I say, 'I will wait till I get into the circumstances then put God to the test,' I shall find I cannot. I must get the thing settled between myself and God...and then I can go forth with the certainty that the battle is won."

Food for Thought
Self-control can't be coerced; it has to be chosen.

A Prayer for Power

Dear God,
Your Word teaches that when we truly experience Your saving grace,
we find the power to say no to wasteful passions
and to live self-controlled and productive lives.
But how much I need Your help
to overcome my laziness and self-deception.
Teach me and change me, Lord.
I want to become more self-controlled.
Today it seems that self-indulgence is the drug of choice on every corner.
But I don't want my appetites to dominate my life!
You promise to live powerfully through me
so that I might love You and serve others.
Now show me how to build the walls of self-control and restraint
around my life.
I relinquish my rebellious will,
which would rob me of the self-control You want me to choose.
Thank You that You are able and willing
to help me today.
Amen.

24 | Take Each Bite with Gladness

He makes grass grow for the cattle, and plants for man to cultivate—bringing forth food from the earth: wine that gladdens the heart of man, oil to make his face shine, and bread that sustains his heart.

PSALM 104:14-15

Not only did God think up the whole idea of food, He actually intended that it be a good thing! He wanted food not just to keep us alive, but also to "gladden" us and to "sustain" us. God never intended for food to become your best friend or your path to fulfillment. But He also never intended for food to become your enemy.

In fact, one surefire way to blow a diet plan is to ban your favorite foods. "The key to losing weight is cutting fat and calories where it hurts the least," says registered dietician Connie Diekman, also a spokesperson for the American Dietetic Association. Quoted in *Heart and Soul* magazine, she advises, "If you love pizza, it's not the food to sacrifice. Doing so will only increase your desire for it. Simply eat smaller portions less often and trim fat from your diet where you won't miss it so much."

Ultimately every source of food is a gift, a provision, from God's hand. And when we adopt this attitude of gratitude, we actually defuse food's power over us. Think of it this way: We don't abuse what we're thankful for. We abuse what we're angry at ourselves for wanting in the first place.

Today take each bite with gladness and with the knowledge that God is the source of all life and the giver of every good gift.

Food for Thought
Food is a gift to receive with gratefulness, not with greed.

A Prayer for Power

Thank You, God,
for giving us food of all kinds,
shapes, colors, aromas, textures, and flavors.
I praise You for strawberries!
And I delight in crisp yellow peppers and juicy oranges!
I praise You for giving us taste buds—
You didn't have to do that!
I praise You also for those edible pleasures
that I sometimes abuse.
Today I ask for the grace
to appreciate the daily sustenance You give me
and to appreciate it so much that I don't feel the need to be greedy.
Maker of everything delicious,
all day long I will notice Your genius and generosity,
and I will honor You with my appetites and my attitude.
Amen.

25 | Blessed Are the Beggars

A blind man, Bartimaeus...was sitting by the roadside begging.... He began to shout, "Jesus, Son of David, have mercy on me!" Many rebuked him and told him to be quiet, but he shouted all the more.... "What do you want me to do for you?" Jesus asked him. The blind man said, "Rabbi, I want to see." "Go," said Jesus, "your faith has healed you." Immediately he received his sight and followed Jesus along the road.

MARK 10:46-52

Bartimaeus could not make his way through the crowds, rush up to Jesus, and ask to be healed. All he could do was sit on the side of the road—blind, begging, and waiting.

Sometimes the journey toward healthy living feels this way. We wait for change; we wait for Jesus to come by and heal us. But in the midst of this waiting and these feelings of want, we have an opportunity that's easy to miss: We can begin to understand what it means to be "poor in spirit."

In *When the Heart Waits,* Sue Monk Kidd writes, "Jesus seemed to have a soft spot for the marginal people of life, including beggars.... Could it be because beggars know how to open their hands, trusting that the crumbs of grace will fall?... A beggar must simply trust, moment by moment.... She lives not with clenched fists but with palms open, ready to receive."

Jesus said, "Blessed are the poor in spirit, for theirs is the kingdom of heaven" (Matt. 5:3). Jesus is going to come by today. Wait for Him, watch for Him as a beggar would, and open your hands to receive His riches.

Food for Thought
Jesus came to feed beggars.

A Prayer for Power

Dear Lord,
how glad I am that You stopped for beggars!
I know what it is to wait for You
and to call out to You for help.
Thank You that You hear every plea
and that Your mercy passes no one by,
not even me!
Today I will wait for You
here by the side of the road.
I will call out for You, with my hands open,
ready to receive Your grace,
Your touch, Your healing.
Jesus, Son of God, have mercy on me!
Amen.

26 | A Busy Body

But you, lazybones, how long will you sleep? When will you wake up?

PROVERBS 6:9, NLT

Most of us would not describe ourselves as idle or lazy. We work hard, either on the job or at home, and chances are we fall into bed exhausted at night. But is it the *right* kind of tired?

Health experts unanimously agree that physical exercise not only boosts our metabolism rate and burns calories, but it also gives us more energy and improves our disposition and mood. And yet only one-fifth of America's adults spend leisure time in a physical activity. One-fourth are completely inactive, and the rest are considered "inadequately active" by the U.S. Centers for Disease Control.

It's true that there will be no stair steppers in heaven. And God will love us the same whether we go to the gym today or not. But He does care about our physical health and our disposition. As Karen Kingsbury writes in *The Prism Weight-Loss Program,* "Don't you think thirty minutes on a treadmill might help ease depression on a day filled with the blues?"

The answer is, "Of course!"

If you haven't already, find the kind of physical activity that you really *enjoy*—and get your body busy feeling better.

Food for Thought
The best way to gain energy is to spend it in the right ways.

62

A Prayer for Power

Dear God,
I don't want to be a lazybones!
Please forgive me for those times
when I fail to keep the body You gave me in good shape.
Thank You for giving me muscles,
and breath,
and the ability to dance, walk, and swim.
Thank You for the gift of exercise
and for all its benefits.
Help me not to neglect this precious gift.
It takes work, Lord.
And sweat.
It's hard some days to get motivated
But Lord of my body,
today I choose to follow You
and to do what is hard.
I ask You to bless my efforts.
Empower me when I am weak,
inspire me when I lose sight of the goal,
and help me to *enjoy* the gift of movement.
Amen.

27 | Soul Wounds

See, the former things have taken place, and new things I declare;
before they spring into being I announce them to you.

ISAIAH 42:9

We've all heard it said, "The past is the past." But often those "former things" have a way of becoming formidable things in our present. Like broken branches fallen across our path, old hurts and memories can block us even as we try to move forward.

Maybe you suffered deep wounding at the hands of family or friends. Maybe you were physically mistreated or sexually abused. Maybe you were verbally injured or abandoned by a parent. Whenever we set about to change our lives from the inside out, these "soul wounds" tend to make themselves felt. Perhaps you used food for years to smother your emotional hurts, and now, when you remove this "anesthesia," you find yourself aching inside.

God can and will heal your wounds. He is doing something new in you! Keep in mind that He often chooses to work through people here on earth who can wrap their arms around you or listen to you. If you need help, seek it. And remember God's tenderness: "A bruised reed he will not break, and a smoldering wick he will not snuff out" (Isa. 42:3).

Food for Thought
Don't let the past trip your present.

A Prayer for Power

Dear God,
You are Lord of my past,
Lord of my present,
and Lord of my future.
Even before I knew You,
You knew me and loved me.
Every hurt I've ever suffered, You saw.
Every tear I've cried, You wanted to wipe away.
Today I ask that You would reveal to me
any hurt or event or piece of my history
that needs Your healing touch.
Show me where there is unforgiveness in my heart.
Show me where I need to look back
in order to see more clearly the way ahead.
By Your power at work in me,
I know I can find the road to victory,
the path to a better present,
and the hope of freedom in my future.
I will look and listen for Your miracle all day!
Amen.

28 | Eve's Dieting Tips

When the woman saw that the fruit of the tree was good for food and pleasing to the eye, and also desirable for gaining wisdom, she took some and ate it.

GENESIS 3:6

Isn't it ironic that it was a woman eating food she shouldn't have that caused the "fall" of humankind? In Eve's mistakes, we can recognize some of our own. For example, just because something is edible doesn't mean it's "good for food." God clearly told Eve, *This is not good for food! In fact, if you eat it, you'll die!*

Her mistake was that she let her eyes do her thinking. She thought the fruit was "pleasing to the eye." Translate this "YUMMY!" In fact, the fruit looked so delicious that she found a way to justify eating it. How? By buying the serpent's lie that it was "desirable for gaining wisdom." What gave her "wisdom," of course, wasn't the fruit, but her own decision to sin.

Likewise, how often have you and I been duped into thinking that food has power that it doesn't? Power to comfort, power to cheer us up, power to make us feel something we're lacking?

If Eve were here today, her top dieting tips might go something like this:

- Don't eat what God says is bad for you.
- Don't gaze too long at the cheesecake.
- Don't seek from food—or anything else—what only God can give.

Food for Thought
Age-old mistakes can be avoided.

A Prayer for Power

Dear God,
I know that I have told myself lies
when I wanted something that You've warned against.
Today I pray for a heart that is surrendered to You.
You alone know what is best for me.
Right now I invite You to show me
what is truly "good for food,"
what will look "pleasing to the eye"—
even after it's on my body.
Reveal to me what life choices will safely lead me
into Your wisdom and truth.
Amen.

29 | Barbie Bondage

All who make idols are nothing, and the things they treasure are worthless. Those who would speak up for them are blind; they are ignorant, to their own shame.

ISAIAH 44:9

An idol is anything we worship above or in place of God. In today's world we make idols of movie and music stars and size-two models, among others. There's nothing wrong with admiring beauty or talent. But when these values, rather than God's values, drive us, we've begun to practice idolatry.

One reason God condemns idolatry is because He knows it will hurt *us.* The phrase "ignorant to their own shame" well describes the woman trapped in "Barbie bondage," idolizing a false image of beauty.

In *You Are Not What You Weigh,* Lisa Bevere writes about Barbie bondage:

> This image is never what we are and is always just beyond our reach.... She is an image molded and forged by the spirit of this world. What she doesn't have, plastic surgery readily supplies. Even this computer generation...reduces her thighs and cinches her waist while sweeping away any sign of imperfection in her skin. She is a deaf, dumb, and blind idol.

When you consider your physical self, refuse to set goals dictated by a false standard that no woman can meet. Seek your reflection in God's eyes alone, and let Him mold you into the beautiful image you see there.

Food for Thought
Admire what's beautiful, but worship the One who created beauty.

A Prayer for Power

Dear God,
please forgive me for wanting to become a fantasy,
an image created by this world,
instead of the real me created by You.
I do not want to worship human beauty.
I want to worship You alone.
I want to set my eyes on You
and to seek to become like You in every way.
Even now, Lord, You say I am beautiful.
When You look at me, You see Your perfect Son,
and all my flaws are eclipsed by His radiance.
Thank You, God, for the beauty that abounds in this world.
Thank You for uniquely feminine beauty, too.
Please help me to respond rightly to every lovely image.
May I admire all that is lovely in this world,
without worshiping it,
without coveting it,
without letting idolatry belittle my soul.
Beautiful Lord,
maker of everything truly beautiful,
I worship and serve You alone.
Amen.

30 | Escape Routes

No temptation has seized you except what is common to man. And God is faith-
ful; he will not let you be tempted beyond what you can bear. But when you are
tempted, he will also provide a way out so that you can stand up under it.

1 CORINTHIANS 10:13

When you sign up for any kind of change, you sign up for a battle. But if
God heads up your plan of attack, it's a battle you can win! God has
promised that He will never tempt us beyond what we can bear and that
He will always provide a way out.

Gwen Shamblin takes this promise literally. "When I know I am not
hungry and just want to eat anyway," she writes in *The Weigh Down Diet*,
"then one of the ingeniously creative things God does is to provide me
with an escape route. My job is to be alert and take advantage of it! At first,
you may not even recognize that God just helped you until after the fact.
But you will become more skilled and more observant as time goes on."

Shamblin lists several different kinds of "escapes." You're about to eat
what or when you shouldn't, but then you're distracted by something else,
or you're disgusted by something wrong with your food, or your food is
"dislocated"—you can't get to it. The small interruption gives you just
enough time to get with God and regroup.

Food for Thought
With God's help, no temptation is unbearable or unbeatable.

A Prayer for Power

Dear God,
save me from defeat!
Don't let temptations trap me today.
When something wrong begins to look good,
help me not to compromise an inch!
Thank You that when I choose to submit my whole heart to You,
I gain power over temptations.
You live inside of me, and You are greater and stronger
than any outer or inner enemy I face.
Instead of succumbing to temptations,
each day I will stay alert to my weaknesses.
And when I'm tempted,
I will look for the way of escape You promise to provide.
With Your help, and by Your power and provision,
I can—and will!—overcome.
Amen.

31 | Thin Happy

*But seek first his kingdom and his righteousness, and all these things
will be given to you as well.*

MATTHEW 6:33

According to *Life* magazine, the average female model weighs 20 percent
less than the average woman, and 85 percent of all American women
weigh more than that model. We envy these ultrathin beauties, but as Lisa
Grunwald points out in *Life,* "You can find a lot of thin, gorgeous bulim-
ics who are as crazy as bedbugs."

Bulimia is a serious disease, and women who suffer from it are not
"crazy." But the point is well-taken: *Thin* and *happy* are not synonyms.
Healthy eating and regular exercise will make you feel a lot better and lift
your spirits, but being physically fit won't change your spiritual inclina-
tions, make you more loving, fill a void in your soul, or cause you to think
of others before yourself.

The real key to happiness? Seeking God and His purposes for your life
above all else. Put Him first, love Him most, seek His principles for living, and care passionately about what He cares about. Then sit back and
watch true happiness bloom.

Food for Thought
Getting thin is not the key to getting happy.

A Prayer for Power

Dear God,
today I realize there are
so many things I seek first in place of You:
I seek to reach *my* goals.
I seek to feel good when I look in the mirror.
I seek to impress people.
I seek to prosper financially.
I seek to enjoy my leisure time.
I seek to feel loved.
Lord, show me today how to truly seek You *first*—
and above all else.
May Your goals become my goals.
May Your concerns become my concerns.
May I earnestly seek to know You
and love You
and worship You—
above all else.
For Your kingdom, God,
is not about eating and drinking,
but about righteousness and peace and *joy*
in Your Holy Spirit (Rom. 14:17).
Amen.

32 | The Powerlessness of Will Power

He that soweth to his flesh shall of the flesh reap corruption; but he that soweth to the Spirit shall of the Spirit reap life everlasting.

GALATIANS 6:8, KJV

Richard Foster writes in *Celebration of Discipline:*

> Our ordinary method of dealing with ingrained sin is to launch a frontal attack. We rely on our will power and determination. Whatever the issue for us may be—anger, bitterness, gluttony, pride, sexual lust, alcohol, fear—we determine never to do it again.... [But] the will has the same deficiency as the law—it can deal only with externals.... When we despair of gaining inner transformation through human powers of will and determination, we are open to a wonderful new realization: inner righteousness is a gift from God to be graciously received. The needed change within us is God's work, not ours.

So does this mean we can sit back, snack on chips, and wait for God to change us? Not at all. Our role is to participate in spiritual disciplines, such as prayer, meditation, Scripture reading. This is how we make ourselves available to God so He can perform His transforming work.

Says Foster, "A farmer is helpless to grow grain; all he can do is to provide the right conditions for the growing of grain." Rather than sow in "the flesh," through your will power, work on creating the right conditions for God to sow the seeds of change in your heart. Open your spirit to His transforming grace, and changes will begin to happen!

Food for Thought
We choose; God changes.

A Prayer for Power

Dear God,
I see it! I see it!
I so often strive in my own strength,
not even realizing that I'm relying on sheer determination,
imagining that what matters most is my own will power.
How ridiculous!
I can't change this heart of mine,
which is deceptive beyond understanding.
But I can offer my heart to You.
I can place my heart under Your care
and expose it to Your power and grace.
I can exercise self-control,
and I can make my spiritual disciplines a top priority.
This is what I want to do!
Please, Lord, forgive my flimsy attempts
at winning with my puny human will power.
Empower me instead with Your inexhaustible power,
which has no limits, no wrong motives, no capacity for deception.
I am Yours.
I will work to make my heart a fertile place
where changes can take deep root
and where real growth has a real chance.
Thank You, God!
Amen.

33 | Comfort Food

Praise be to...the Father of compassion and the God of all comfort,
who comforts us in all our troubles.

2 CORINTHIANS 1:3-4

When Sasha, a high-powered attorney in New York, lost a big client the same week her mother died, she turned to food for comfort. "I gorged myself," she says, "on all those 'comfort foods' like pasta, mashed potatoes, and ice cream.... But the weight I gained made me even more depressed. It took me several months to retrain my mind and my stomach and get back on track."

Sasha's is a common scenario. "Circumstances may be spinning out of control," writes Karen Kingsbury in *The Prism Weight-Loss Program.* "Chaos may rein, but if we can get to our stash of comfort food, we can dim the effect...and trick ourselves into believing that all is right with the world."

God, the Comforter, has a better answer. The reason we are tempted to indulge any addiction is usually to dull some inner pain. Next time you feel weak and something inside hurts, STOP. Ask God specifically to comfort you. It may not happen that very second, but if you wait on Him, His Holy Spirit will fill you with peace and satisfaction.

Food for Thought
Make God's presence your comfort food.

A PRAYER FOR POWER

God of all comfort,
You alone know all the times I have been hurting,
and You have been there—
loving me, listening to me, touching me with gentle healing.
You know about those wounds and sorrows
that go so deep I sometimes can't even name them.
That is why I praise You—
because You are what You say: the God of all comfort!
No one else could reach inside my heart
and strengthen me the way You do.
Because You comfort me,
I don't have to use food, sex, or drugs destructively
in order to dull my pain.
Today I choose, so far as it is possible for me, Lord,
to turn to You when I'm hurting,
and I ask You to carry me in Your arms of compassion and strength.
Thank You, God, for loving me so tenderly.
Amen.

34 | Dressing-Room Lies

I praise you because I am fearfully and wonderfully made.

PSALM 139:14

When was the last time you thought, *I am wonderfully made!* When was the last time you talked about yourself this way to others?

It probably wasn't while you were trying on clothes in a dressing room.

The truth is, if we were to suddenly actually *become* what we say about ourselves, most of us would be horrified by what we saw.

In her book *7 Ways to Build a Better You,* Sheri Rose Shepherd writes:

> I remember being with my mother in the dressing room. To me, my mother was the most beautiful woman in the world. I would watch her try on clothes, and I'd say, "Mommy, you look so beautiful!"
>
> She'd roll her eyes and say, "Oh, I look horrible in this! I look fat! Look at what this is doing to me!"
>
> I remember thinking, "Wow! I can't wait to do that! I will grow up and try on things and when someone tells me I look beautiful, I'll say, 'I'm disgusting! I'm fat! I'm gross!' "

Like Sheri, many of us grew up being trained to talk negatively about our bodies. But when we do so, we are putting down God's creation, acting as our own worst enemy, and setting a bad example. The good news is that it's never too late to change. Listen to yourself carefully today. Compliment yourself. Let God lift your chin, look into your eyes, and say, "You are wonderfully made!" Hear His words. He's telling the truth!

Food for Thought
I am wonderfully made!

A Prayer for Power

Dear God,
deposit this truth in the deepest pockets of my heart:
I am wonderfully made because I was made by You.
And not only was I made by You,
I was redeemed by You!
I have been remade, recreated, and spiritually reconfigured
so that I am becoming more and more like Your Son.
Show me how to speak well, Lord,
of all that You created in Your genius and love.
Help me to humbly tell the truth:
I am Yours, and, therefore, I am of great worth.
My body is precious and good
because it houses Your Spirit.
My mind is of great value
because it is being renewed daily by You.
My heart and spirit are miracles
because they are Your workmanship.
This is why I choose today
to stop beating myself up
and to celebrate the beauty of Your handiwork.
Amen.

35 | Romanced by God

No longer will they call you Deserted, or name your land Desolate. But you will be called Hephzibah, and your land Beulah.... As a bridegroom rejoices over his bride, so will your God rejoice over you.

Isaiah 62:4-5

Do you ever think of God as your lover or husband? Throughout the Bible, God repeatedly compares His love for Israel and later, for the church, to a husband's love for his bride. Many believe that the entire book of Song of Songs is a metaphor for God's passionate pursuit of a people He adores.

In Isaiah, God expresses His love for Israel by telling her that though she's been "Deserted" and "Desolate," He is now going to call her Hephzibah, meaning "my delight is in her," and "Beulah," which means "married."

When a woman knows that she is loved by a man, her entire being shines with the assurance that she's wanted and adored. God wants you to have that same assurance—from Him. No earthly love can compare! Your beau may leave you desolate. Your husband could desert you physically or emotionally. But God's love for you never will fall short.

At this very moment can you feel Him rejoicing over you? He is passionate about you! You are a delight to His eyes—just as you are. You are precious in His sight.

Food for Thought
People will fail you, but God is faithful forever.

A PRAYER FOR POWER

Dear God,
do You really love me like a devoted husband?
It is comforting to know that You are jealous for me,
that You are devoted to me,
that You have a covenant with me that is stronger
than any earthly marriage.
Thank You that when I experience Your love,
I have so much more love to share with others.
I want to shine today
with the assurance of Your faithfulness to me.
In all my efforts to transform myself physically,
I know that the most beautifying thing I can do is to remember
that You are rejoicing over me.
I praise You that You will not leave me desolate,
but will embrace me—just as I am—from this day forward.
Amen.

36 | Holy Beauty

*He had no beauty or majesty to attract us to him, nothing in his appearance
that we should desire him. He was despised and rejected by men, a man of
sorrows, and familiar with suffering. Like one from whom men hide their faces
he was despised, and we esteemed him not.*

ISAIAH 53:2-3

Isaiah's prophetic description of Jesus is disconcerting, isn't it? Contrary to
the lovely, haloed Jesus so often depicted by artists, the Bible tells us that
"he had no beauty." The Hebrew word for *beauty* here is the same one
used to describe David (1 Sam. 16:18) and is translated "fine-looking."
Jesus had none of David's legendary handsomeness. He had *no beauty*. He
wasn't esteemed. He was rejected and despised unto death.

That about sums up our greatest fears for ourselves, doesn't it?

Yet, Paul writes, "Your attitude should be the same as that of Christ
Jesus: Who…made himself nothing" (Phil. 2:5-7). This is God's goal for
you: to be conformed to Christ's likeness (Rom. 8:29).

What does this say about efforts to improve our appearance? Are they
all wrong? Should we aim to be ugly, fat, and rejected?

No. We do not sin if we are attractive any more than we become holy
by neglecting our appearance. However, if we are obsessed with gaining
acceptance, admirable glances, and the envy and esteem of friends, we are
radically off track and, in truth, not interested in becoming like Jesus at all.

To truly seek to be like Christ is to choose humility over pride, growth
over comfort, God's approval over people's, and the beauty of holiness
over the fleeting beauty of our physical frame.

Food for Thought
Admire the One who had no beauty.

A Prayer for Power

Dear God,
when I remember Your suffering,
the rejection You endured, the shame You embraced,
I am appalled at myself.
I am so shallow, Lord.
I confess that I want to be accepted, admired, esteemed.
But do I want these things more than I want to be like You?
No, I don't!
Take this small, human heart of mine
and transform it by Your Spirit.
Who am I to expect or long for what You Yourself were denied?
Rescue me from my petty, shortsighted pride and arrogance.
Show me how to empty myself,
to be humble,
to seek Your admiration, not this world's.
Open my spiritual eyes
so that I will recognize, long for, and fight to attain true beauty.
Beauty made perfect by suffering and sacrifice.
Beauty beyond compare.
Holy beauty that is You.
Amen.

37 | Son-Bathing

God is love. Whoever lives in love lives in God, and God in him.

1 JOHN 4:16

It sounds like a slogan from the '70s Jesus Movement. But the phrase "God is love" comes straight from Scripture and is as true today as when the apostle John first wrote it (presumably not on the side of a Volkswagen bus).

But how is it that these three simple words can be so hard to grasp where it counts—in the heart? How does one *live in God's love?*

One way is through prayer. Not the kind where you're reeling off requests, but the kind where you're simply quiet, aware of God within and around you. You can do this while you're driving, while you're cooking, even while you're exercising. As you bask in His presence, you bask in love.

Brennan Manning writes in *Lion and Lamb:*

> The most important thing that ever happens in prayer is letting ourselves be loved by God.... Prayer is like sun bathing. When you spend a lot of time in the sun, people notice it. You look like you've been out in the sun because you've got a tan. Prayer—or bathing in the Son of God's love (Son-bathing?)—makes you look different. The awareness of being loved brings a lightness and a tint of brightness and sometimes, for no apparent reason, a smile plays at the corner of your mouth.

Next time you're tempted to look for love in the kitchen cupboard, spend time basking in the presence of Jesus instead. It's time to start working on that Son-tan—a life of love that shines for all to see.

Food for Thought
Bathe in the light and love of the Son.

A Prayer for Power

Dear God,
I want to bask in Your love!
Why do I ever put it off?
When I finally settle down to just be in Your presence,
I feel Your warm smile upon me.
Rescue me, Lord, from this pale, sickly self
and draw me into the light of Your love.
I want to be a person who loves to rest in Your presence
and has a Son-tan—a life of love—to prove it.
Help me to completely abandon myself to You
and to all the truth You want to shine into my life.
In You there is no darkness, Lord.
What a cure for the blues!
When I'm tempted to look for love in all the wrong places—
like other's approval, in the fridge, or at the gym —
draw me back to You with the truth.
Today by Your power at work in me,
I will lift my face to You,
I will lay my whole life and self before You,
and I will bask in the warmth of Your holy,
radiant love all day.
Amen.

38 | Waste Not, Lose Not

When they had all had enough to eat, [Jesus] said to his disciples, "Gather the pieces that are left over. Let nothing be wasted."

JOHN 6:12

The issue of not wasting food is a challenging one for the careful eater. Many of us remember our mother saying, "Think of the poor people starving around the world!" But the truth of the matter is that if you don't finish everything on your plate, no one is *really* going to ship it off to a famine-plagued country.

Notice that after Jesus fed the five thousand, He *didn't* say, "Make sure to stuff yourselves!" He said, "Let's save the leftovers." The fact is, the Bible never condones eating more than our fill.

But what happens when you're at a restaurant? The servings are heaping, the maître d´ is doting. You paid twenty-five dollars for that prime rib. Now are you going to just waste it by not cleaning your plate?

Yes. And no. Think about it. Which is the greater waste? For that food to turn into another ripple on your thigh or for it to biodegrade in a landfill? Isn't real waste to eat with gluttony what you'll regret later?

Some tips for eating out: Go where you know you'll be served healthy food, eat a salad before you order more (your appetite will have diminished), don't hesitate to split a meal with someone, request a take-home box if appropriate, stop before you're stuffed. And finally, enjoy what you eat!

Food for Thought
Don't let the fear of waste ruin your waist.

A Prayer for Power

Dear God,
You know that I hate to see good food go uneaten.
But I know that this is no excuse to overindulge myself.
When I think about all the excess food,
all the Dumpsters of it our society throws away each day,
I feel sick.
Lord, with every bite I take, teach me to be grateful.
Today I remember in prayer all those around the world
whom my mother used to worry about.
I pray that there would be a growing awareness in me—
and among all those who are trying to eat less—
that while we live in excess and plenty,
millions live in want, hunger, and desperate need.
Move us to action, Lord.
Even as I choose not to waste food by eating more than I need,
I choose to do something for those who can't imagine leftovers,
much less a dilemma such as dieting.
Help me to think rightly, God—
to have the right perspective on these and other food issues
and to take one step today to make a difference in the world.
Amen.

39 | Hunger Pangs

Man shall not live by bread alone, but by every word that proceedeth out of the mouth of God.

MATTHEW 4:4, KJV

Are you starving your spirit to spite your soul?

We live in such a physical world, and when we focus on transforming our physical bodies, we can neglect the deep hunger of our souls. If we don't "eat" enough of God's Word or if we don't listen for God's voice often enough, we end up feeling empty inside because we're hungry for God.

Of course, some hunger pangs are purely physical in origin. But our most important pangs are intended to call us to our spiritual center, reminding us that ultimately God alone satisfies.

Today estimate how much time you spend buying, helping to prepare, or eating food. Then add up how much time you're spending taking in "the Bread of Life." Which part of you is being stuffed, and which is being starved?

Food for Thought
Ask: Is that my stomach growling or my soul?

A PRAYER FOR POWER

Lord,
thank You that You are
"the living bread that came down from heaven"
to give us life.
You said, "If anyone eats of this bread,
he will live forever" (John 6:51).
What a wonderful promise, Lord!
Help me to remember that when I feel
empty or hollow inside
and I am tempted to fill that void inappropriately with food,
You alone are the "bread" I need.
Thank You for Your living water, the Holy Spirit,
who quenches my thirsty soul.
Today may every snack and drink and meal and dessert
remind me how much I also need to feed my spirit
and that every word that comes out of Your mouth
is like gourmet food for my soul.
Amen.

40 | Binge Alert

Do not join those who drink too much wine or gorge themselves on meat.

PROVERBS 23:20

"Gorge" is such an ugly word. "Gluttony"—habitual gorging—is even worse. Until recent times, gluttony was viewed as the privilege of the wealthy and powerful. Caesars, kings, and lords held eating and drinking feasts that could last for weeks. Unbridled excess represented great wealth.

We'd like to deny ever being gluttons. But most of us have eaten or drunk too much—some of us habitually—and we haven't needed a medieval banquet to do it!

Have you ever noticed that after you gorge, you don't really feel satisfied? Instead, you feel like a grossly overstuffed failure. There are physical reasons for the missing payoff. According to Gwen Shamblin, author of *The Weigh Down Diet,* as you overeat, your taste buds actually lose the ability to taste. "The reason salts and sweets are the typical choice for the binge," she says, "is that the body is full; therefore, the taste buds on the tongue are dulled. As you approach a 2,000 to 10,000 calorie binge, you literally cannot taste anything."

The truth is that when we binge, we're buying a lie. It goes something like: "If I eat like a pig, I must be living like a king." But that's a lie that will make us sick in body *and* spirit.

Better to enjoy the lasting wealth of wise living that fills us with truth, satisfies fully, and leaves no regrets.

Food for Thought
I can best eat my fill when I don't go past full.

A Prayer for Power

Dear God,
right now, I surrender to You my temptation
to binge,
to rebel,
to misuse the food You've blessed me with.
Fill me instead with Your Spirit and grace
and grant me the power
and will to STOP indulging
when my stomach is no longer hungry.
Thank You that by Your Spirit within me,
I have the ability to resist the urge to overeat today.
Amen.

41 | In the Eye of the Beholder

Shall what is formed say to him who formed it, "Why did you make me like this?"

ROMANS 9:20

We live in an age where for the first time women can change their bodies in dramatic ways apart from natural weight loss or exercise. Fat can be sucked out with liposuction. Breasts can be augmented. And not only for adults. According to a recent article in *USA Today*, teenage cosmetic surgeries in the U.S. have nearly doubled.

The issue raises complicated questions. *Where do you draw the line between a defect and a deformity? How is cosmetic surgery different from makeup? When is it calling "bad" what God has created?*

If you or someone you love is considering liposuction or plastic surgery of some kind, here are some questions to consider:

- Is it about vanity, or is it a medical or emotional need?
- Am I trying to look like the glossy media images of "the beautiful people"?
- Have I prayed about this and sought God's and others' counsel?
- Am I trying to take a shortcut to a better body rather than work at it?
- Am I completely aware of the health and safety risks?
- Am I in a position financially to pay for the procedure without shortchanging my commitments to others and to God?

Today meditate on these words: "I praise you because I am fearfully and wonderfully made; your works are wonderful, I know that full well" (Ps. 139:14).

Food for Thought
Shortcuts usually shortchange you.

A Prayer for Power

Dear God,
how easy it is to forget that
You made me.
From scratch. From nothing!
One minute I didn't exist; then I did.
And nothing about my body is an accident.
You planned every part of me.
Forgive me for feeling angry about some of the traits I have.
Help me to change my perspective, God.
Before I consider drastic medical interventions,
help me first learn to accept
and even appreciate my physical characteristics.
You didn't intend for me to look like anyone else!
Today I choose to stop worrying and fussing
about that physical "problem" I focus on so much.
I surrender it to You,
and I open my conscience, understanding, and emotions
to receive Your perfect wisdom for me.
I thank You that I am not what I look like to me.
I am what I look like to You.
Beauty really is in the eye of the Beholder.
Amen.

42 | A Lighter Load

Come to me, all you who are weary and burdened, and I will give you rest.
Take my yoke upon you and learn from me, for I am gentle and humble in
heart, and you will find rest for your souls.

MATTHEW 11:28-29

Do the words "weary" and "burdened" describe the state of your soul today? Maybe you've been on a yo-yo cycle for years and you're just plain tired of working at it. Or perhaps you're weighed down not only by the pounds you want to lose, but by the troubles of this life.

Jesus understands. Listen to His words in *The Message:* "Are you tired? Worn out? Burned out on religion? Come to me. Get away with me and you'll recover your life. I'll show you how to take a real rest. Walk with me and work with me—watch how I do it. Learn the unforced rhythms of grace. I won't lay anything heavy or ill-fitting on you. Keep company with me and you'll learn to live freely and lightly" (Matt. 11:28-30).

Ask yourself: Have I been carrying around a big load of worries? As I work to please God or others, am I shouldering alone the burden of doing things "right" rather than relying on God's power?

Jesus wants to give you rest today. Will you let Him take your heavy load and learn from Him the unforced rhythms of grace? Hear the Lord inviting you today to a place of peace and gentle rest.

Food for Thought
Let Jesus lighten your load.

A Prayer for Power

Dear God,
sometimes I feel as if I'm pedaling a bike
up a hill in the wrong gear.
Lord, You say You understand and want to help.
You watch me with compassion, and You call, "Come to me!"
But so often I ride by, unseeing,
unwilling to believe that You would take
this load of failures and troubles on Your own back
and ride in tandem with me,
making even the hardest uphill paths seem easy.
I want to please You, and I want to obey You.
I want to put forth effort to do what is right.
Show me, Lord, how to work hard
and how to love You with all my heart.
But don't let me ignore Your sweet invitation
to rest,
to peace,
to partner with Your strength
as I go on my way today.
Amen.

43 | Desperate Measures

A simple man believes anything, but a prudent man gives thought to his steps.

PROVERBS 14:15

Sometimes we get so desperate to lose weight that we will believe anything. For example, Oprah Winfrey once set up a phony diet program in a mall to test just how gullible—or desperate—weight-conscious consumers are. The program offered shoppers the Hot Dog Diet. Forty-five customers actually signed up!

Such desperation may seem humorous at first, but it reflects the kind of reckless desire to lose weight that all too often backfires on the earnest dieter.

The Bible tells us that the keys to success are to have a discerning heart that seeks knowledge (Prov. 15:14) and to give careful thought to our efforts (Hag. 1:5). When you're tempted to take desperate measures in your zeal to attain your goals—stop. Don't give in to foolishness. Consult with God about your plans, be open to course corrections, and entrust Him with your agenda—including the timing of the results.

Food for Thought
Desperate measures don't deliver.

A PRAYER FOR POWER

Dear God,
I admit that often I am tempted
to look for a shortcut—
an easier way to get dramatic results.
Sometimes I get so eager to see change
that I take desperate measures
that don't deliver.
Today, because I can count on Your help,
I commit to doing due diligence instead.
Give me perseverance where I am impatient,
grant me strength where I am weak.
Make me desperate only for You!
Make me zealous to take the right steps,
to choose the good course,
to be an example to everyone I meet.
Keep me from foolishness, Lord.
Show me Your way, and I will walk in it.
Amen.

44 | Miss Piggy

Like a gold ring in a pig's snout is a beautiful woman who shows no discretion.

PROVERBS 11:22

Okay, so you've lost some weight, you've been working out, and your body is becoming something you're less ashamed of. In fact, you're sorta proud of it now. Suddenly you can wear tailored clothes and shop anywhere. Suddenly your friends want to look like you…and you notice that men look…

The desire to be admired seems an innocent one, and it may get you started on the road to better health. But if you are motivated by a need for admiration, you've fallen victim to vanity. It's an ugly word, isn't it? Just check out the synonyms: egotistical, inflated, proud, fat-headed.

No one sets out to be vain. However, this desire to flaunt your beauty, whether you've reached your goal or not, can sneak up on you unawares. Vanity easily leads to immodesty—"showing no discretion." We've all observed this attitude in a woman. She's like a pig with a gold ring in her nose, a beautiful woman cheapened by her vanity.

As Sheri Rose Shepherd points out in *7 Ways to Build a Better You,* "[The goal of healthy eating is] not about being Barbie with a Bible. It's not about being in a pageant or being on the cover of *Fit* magazine. It's about presenting your body as a living and holy sacrifice to God."

What could be more lovely than a woman devoted to God above all else who refuses to use her beauty to arouse envy or lust in others?

Food for Thought
Beauty sought for vanity's sake is always sought in vain.

A Prayer for Power

Dear God,
sometimes vanity seems like a monster
I just can't outrun.
It's not that I think I'm beautiful and want to show off.
But I confess I want to be in the position to do that!
Please forgive me for being focused on outward beauty
instead of nurturing the kind of inward loveliness
that You create within those who worship You.
How much brighter is the beauty
that shines out from a heart that reflects Your glory,
not its own!
I humble myself before You, Lord,
and repent of my pride,
my pigheadedness,
my passion to be admired.
Help me to aspire to achieve my goals
for a healthy body and mind,
with the right motives guiding my efforts.
Thank You that You are able to change me—
from the inside out!
Today I will seek *Your* admiration
most of all.
Amen.

45 | The Overweight Church

He who conceals his sins does not prosper, but whoever confesses and renounces them finds mercy.

PROVERBS 28:13

If abusing our bodies with too much food is sinful, then why don't we hear more about this sin at church? We discuss sexual sins, pride, dishonesty, and greed. But when was the last sermon you heard about gluttony?

One reason is that most of these other sins are hidden. You can't glance around the room and see who's "guilty" of lust.

Another reason for the silence, according to Linda S. Mintle, Ph.D., in a *Charisma* magazine article, is that "food indulgence is somewhat sanctioned in the church. Eating is deeply embedded in church culture. We organize, meet, greet, celebrate, study, live and die around food.... Sure, we overeat at the church picnic; but overindulgence with food is not as stigmatized as, say, drunkenness."

Like any kind of behavior that hurts us and grieves God, overeating needs to be addressed. But it should always be treated with tact, and those who struggle in this area deserve compassionate support. Many churches have support groups, such as Overeaters Anonymous. There, those who struggle can confess their failures, experience the mercy God promises, and find the friendship and accountability they need to make changes.

Food for Thought
Church is a place for confession, not covering up;
compassion, not condemnation.

A Prayer for Power

Dear God,
today I pray for all people everywhere
who struggle with overeating.
Have mercy on them, Lord.
Have mercy on me!
Give Your church grace and wisdom to reach out to people
who are caught in a cycle of overeating and underexercising.
May there be no spirit of judgment toward them,
but one of love, mercy, and genuine caring.
Show me how I can reach out
to help others who need support.
May there be no prejudice
in how I treat other fellow strugglers in Your church.
Make us one in You, God, thin and heavy alike.
May we lift one another up in prayer daily
and lift a hand to help whenever we see a need.
Gather to Your heart all who love You
and need Your power at work in them.
Have mercy on us, and forgive us.
Amen.

46 | Fasting from the Heart

But when you fast, put oil on your head and wash your face, so that it will not be obvious to men that you are fasting, but only to your Father, who is unseen; and your Father, who sees what is done in secret, will reward you.

MATTHEW 6:17-18

Have you ever considered fasting—not to lose weight, but to gain greater self-control and increased sensitivity to God?

In *Celebration of Discipline,* Richard Foster says, "More than any other single discipline, fasting reveals the things that control us." As we turn from our physical appetites, we experience a spiritual edge that makes us more attuned to God.

Although Jesus didn't command fasting, we know by His statement "When you fast..." (Matt. 6:16) that He assumed people *would* fast. But He cautioned them not to do it for any external reward.

Foster observes, "At times there is such stress upon the blessings and benefits of fasting, we would be tempted to believe that with a little fast we could have the world, including God, eating out of our hand. Fasting must forever center on God."

Before you embark on a fast, be sure to check with your doctor for guidelines. If you are on a healthy diet program, follow its recommendations. Always drink plenty of fluids, and end your fast with a light meal.

A final thought from Sheri Rose Shepherd's *7 Ways to Build a Better You:* "A diet will change the way you look, but a fast will change the way you live. A diet will change your appearance, but a fast will change the way you see everything."

Food for Thought
When you put yourself in a place of want, you experience God's plenty.

A PRAYER FOR POWER

Dear God,
guide me, speak to me, let me know
when You are nudging me toward a time of fasting.
And when I fast,
may I always have right motives.
May I not rush through it,
or see it as a chance to prove my spirituality to others,
or use it to gain sympathy for my "suffering."
Above all, may I never fast simply to lose weight,
while pretending I am fasting for You.
Fill me with Your wisdom, Lord.
Give me the grace I need to commit
to the kind of spiritual disciplines that put me in a place
where You can change me in significant and eternal ways.
I want to be a candidate for that kind of transformation!
I want to experience Your resurrection power,
to be brought back to life because I choose to die
to self and my raging appetites.
As I put myself in a place of want and hunger,
I know that You will meet me there
to sustain me, speak to me, and—as you choose—
miraculously transform me.
Amen.

47 | Feeling Green

A heart at peace gives life to the body, but envy rots the bones.

PROVERBS 14:30

It's been said that women don't dress (and diet, and spend oodles on makeup) for men but for other women. Obviously, this isn't always the case. But it is true that fierce unspoken competition often takes place among women. And the arena of weight loss and fitness is prime breeding ground for such jealousy and striving.

Angela, a petite twenty-something, confesses: "When my best friend Kim went from a size twelve to an eight, and I had to listen to everybody telling her how great she looked, it irked me a bit. I felt betrayed somehow. Even though I'd always disdained diets, I embarked on one with a fury, though quietly, privately. I didn't want anyone to guess the truth: I couldn't stand for my best friend to look better than me."

Envy might spark some right actions you've been putting off, but it's certainly not the kind of inspiration that leads to healthy, permanent changes in lifestyle. The opposite of jealousy is a "heart at peace." Whereas jealousy is like a disease that rots us from the inside out, a heart at peace is life enhancing.

If you realize that you struggle with jealousy, ask God to help you turn that envy into admiration for His creation. Confess your wrong attitudes, and reach out today to receive the ultimate antidote: a heart at peace in the security and nurture of Christ's love.

Food for Thought
Jealousy spoils everything.

A PRAYER FOR POWER

Dear God,
I really do want a heart that is at peace!
I admit that the tentacles of envy
grab hold of me from time to time.
And sometimes I let them wrap their slimy arms
so tightly around my heart
that I covet other women's beauty.
I envy and resent that friend
who doesn't have to worry about what she eats.
You are right, Lord,
that when I allow these feelings a firm grip on my heart,
when I nurse them and use them to motivate me,
they sabotage me sooner or later.
I get angry and think:
It's not fair! I can't be somebody else! I can only be me!
You know all this. And You care.
Thank You, God, for caring!
Forgive me of all pride and selfishness.
Set me free today from any attitudes that would "rot my bones."
Fill me with Your Spirit instead.
And may my heart be at peace in Your loving presence.
Amen.

48 | Fat and Happy?

A happy heart makes the face cheerful, but heartache crushes the spirit.

PROVERBS 15:13

In recent years several celebrity women and the media have bandied the idea that it's possible to be fat and happy. It's true! Heavy people should be no less happy than thin people. In fact, women who are happy have a much better chance of losing weight than women who are miserable.

However, if we take "fat and happy" to mean "I don't care one iota how heavy I get," that's another matter. There's a big difference between being "fat" in the unhealthy, obese sense and being perfectly healthy but large. Obesity is usually defined as a weight 20 percent above normal or as a body-fat proportion above 30 percent for women and 25 percent for men.

In *The Prism Weight-Loss Program*, Karen Kingsbury points out the dangers of obesity:

> It's been said that some of the most dangerous weapons in our society today are the knife and fork. The facts back that up: There are a myriad of serious physical problems—some of them life threatening—associated with excess weight. Cardiovascular disease, hypertension, several types of cancer, diabetes, and problems in the joints and bones.... The latest statistics indicate that obesity is second only to smoking as a contributing factor in illness and premature death.

If you're tempted to participate in the "fat and happy" philosophy for yourself or another, take a second look. And ask if true happiness might be found in true healthiness.

Food for Thought
Trade in "fat and happy" for "fit and healthy."

A Prayer for Power

Dear God,
thank You that You intend for all people—
no matter what their weight—
to be happy and to rejoice in the gift of life.
I know, however,
that being very heavy is a great burden,
that it causes all kinds of practical hassles,
not to mention myriad health risks.
I want to take to heart these truths, Lord.
Help me to think correctly about obesity
and to always make matters of health a priority.
Today I pray for obese women everywhere,
who feel shunned or unloved,
who are unhappy, even miserable because of their weight.
Send all of us help, Lord.
May we find our way to freedom!
Thank You that You love me no matter what.
Thank You that with Your help,
I can learn to eat and live in a way
that pleases me as much as it pleases You.
Amen.

49 | The Lies We Tell Ourselves

The tongue that brings healing is a tree of life, but a deceitful tongue crushes the spirit.

PROVERBS 15:4

We all know that lying to people is wrong. But what about lying to ourselves? When the truth hurts, it's no wonder we'd rather protect ourselves. Do you recognize yourself in this passage from Karen Kingsbury's *The Prism Weight-Loss Program*?

> Food addicts lie to themselves about the way they look and about what and how much they eat.... If you are twenty pounds overweight, you may have convinced yourself that if you dress a certain way no one will really notice and that you can continue overeating. A closet full of long, dark jackets and black slacks will cover just about any problem, you tell yourself.... You look in the mirror each day and assure yourself that you certainly could be worse off. Then you work to think of someone who is fatter than you. This is the way many of us have rationalized our weight for years and years.

As long as we deceive ourselves about our problems, we can't resolve them. We actually "crush" our own spirit.

But here's the good news: There's a part of you, the best and holy part of you, that's tired of being lied to. She has a healing tongue, not a deceitful one. Today invite her and God into the hidden corners of your heart, and invite them to tell you nothing but the whole truth.

Food for Thought
The most damaging lies are those I tell myself.

A Prayer for Power

Dear God,
right now I feel as if You've
turned on a light in my soul,
and I don't like what I see there.
Crouching in the shadows are wimpy lies,
half-truths, rationalizations, and even a few humongous whoppers.
Have I really been so blind?
Forgive me.
Take my hand, Lord, and help me
look at myself and face the truth—
the whole, unattractive truth.
I know that because You are by my side,
not only can I bear to face it,
I can respond to the truth with grace.
But I need to feel Your mercies, God,
if I'm going to admit these inadequacies,
these seemingly hopeless weaknesses that hold sway in my deepest heart.
Right now I pledge to come clean.
I invite the search, and I welcome the sacred part of me,
the part that lives by the power of Your Spirit,
to tell me the truth today.
I'm listening, Lord.
Amen.

50 | Little Sister

We have a young sister, and her breasts are not yet grown.

Song of Songs 8:8

Grown women aren't the only ones confronted with false beauty standards in the media. Every day girls from eight to eighteen receive warped messages about beauty, sexuality, and what it means to be healthy.

The damage is staggering. Up to 10 percent of high school and college students are estimated to have eating disorders such as bulimia, anorexia nervosa, and a newly defined one known as binge eating (bulimia without purging). Studies suggest the death rate for such victims may be as high as 18 percent.

You may or may not have a younger sister or a daughter. But in one sense, we all do: the young girls we meet at church, those who baby-sit for us, those who are eavesdropping in the next dressing room. Often we don't realize that we are sending a message, but we are.

Lisa Bevere writes in *You Are Not What You Weigh*, "I hear a lot of moms say, 'I don't understand why my twelve-year-old daughter is worrying about dieting.' Well, you may never have said anything to her about dieting, but she hears what you say about yourself."

It may seem a small thing, but it's not. Watch what you say. Make it a point whenever possible to tell a young girl you know how lovely she is. But don't just focus on her looks. Tell her if she's funny or smart or discerning. Tell her the truth about drastic measures and eating disorders. And by all means, tell her what you wish someone would have told you.

Food for Thought
The next generation is listening.

A Prayer for Power

Dear God,
today I pray for all those young girls
who are soaking up harmful ideas
about beauty, their bodies, and their worth.
Send messengers of truth their way, Lord!
And let me be one of them.
Make me more conscious of the way I talk,
the way I primp,
the remarks I make.
By Your power at work in me,
help me to refrain from putting myself or my body down.
May I hold my tongue,
arrest my thoughts,
and speak something that builds up instead.
Thank You that every daughter of Yours
is precious in Your eyes.
I know You have made each one lovely
in her own way.
And I choose today to help You, God,
to let every sister of mine and daughter of Yours
know that she is celebrated and adored by You.
Amen.

51 | Mercy Every Moment

For we do not have a high priest who is unable to sympathize with our weaknesses, but we have one who has been tempted in every way, just as we are—yet was without sin. Let us then approach the throne of grace with confidence, so that we may receive mercy and find grace to help us in our time of need.

HEBREWS 4:15-16

This passage is one of the most comforting and promising in Scripture. And it's also one of the most important keys to personal change.

So often we imagine that we must defeat temptation on our own. We battle with sin, and then if we win, we feel okay to approach God. If we lose, we imagine that the next time God sees us coming, He'll say, "You again? You did *what* again?"

But just the opposite is true! Jesus wants you to unabashedly approach Him for help *even while you're in the grip* of excruciating temptation. He won't shun you or be disgusted by you. He understands exactly what you're going through!

Remember, it wasn't Satan who led Jesus out to the desert to be tempted but the Spirit of God (Matt. 4:1). Jesus was "tempted in every way, just as we are" so we could trust Him in our many times of need. What a relief! What freedom!

Meditate all day long on these three key words from today's scripture: *Mercy. Grace. Help.* They're gifts Jesus wants to give you—and they're available at the exact moment when you need them most.

Food for Thought
There is no way to make Jesus turn away.

A Prayer for Power

Dear Lord Jesus,
my heart heaves a great sigh of relief
as I try to take all this in:
There is no darkness in me so thick
that Your love can fail to penetrate it.
There is no temptation in me so ugly
that You don't recognize and conquer it on sight.
There is no failure in my life so complete
that You don't have grace to cover it.
There is no way
I can make You turn away.
Your grace is too great for me to fathom!
Only You know how much I need Your help.
Only You know how scheming and weak I really am.
Have mercy on me, Jesus.
Strengthen and help me in my time of need,
give me grace in my hour of temptation,
be my brother and high priest when I fail.
Amen.

52 | It's All in Your Head

Finally, brothers, whatever is true, whatever is noble, whatever is right, whatever is pure, whatever is lovely, whatever is admirable—if anything is excellent or praiseworthy—think about such things.

PHILIPPIANS 4:8

In *The Prism Weight-Loss Program,* Karen Kingsbury writes about defeatist thinking: "The average diet lasts just four days because people allow their minds to entertain wrong thoughts. Sometimes we actually invite them into our minds, putting them up as regular houseguests. This self-defeating habit must be done away with if you are to find lasting success."

The old cliche "garbage in, garbage out" could also read "wrong thoughts in, diet success out." But here's the good news: We can change the way we think! One way to flush out the negative thoughts that lead to defeat is to focus on truths found in God's Word. Another way is to spend time with the One who "thinks" only the truth.

God knows that what we spend time taking into our minds will affect what makes itself at home in our heart. "Set your mind on things above, not on earthly things," wrote Paul (Col. 3:2). In other words, "Get your nose out of the fashion magazine and off the TV stars and look at Jesus." In order to "have the mind of Christ" (1 Cor. 2:16), we must have Christ on our minds.

As Gwen Shamblin writes in *The Weigh Down Diet,* "We must behold Christ.... If we behold or adore food, we will become a refrigerator. If we behold and adore Christ, we will become like Christ."

What do you want to become? Think on, behold, treasure these things.

Food for Thought
Think about who you want to become.

A Prayer for Power

Dear God,
if I could physically remove my mind
and just hand it over to You,
I would.
But it's not that easy.
You want me to set my thoughts
by my own volition and choice
on what is right and good and pure and true.
That is You!
Today I choose to do just that.
Grant me the will and the power, Lord,
to behold You all day long
as I go about my work and routines.
Thank You that You are indeed
changing me from the inside out
and that as I focus my thoughts on You,
I become more and more like You.
Because of Your mighty power at work in my weakness,
I know I have all the strength I need
to overcome temptations,
to resist self-indulgence,
to do what I truly want to do:
obey and love You.
Amen.

53 | Do I Look Fat in This?

An honest answer is like a kiss on the lips.

PROVERBS 24:26

If an honest answer is like a kiss on the lips, friends and relatives of the dieter might say, "An honest *question* is like a kiss on the lips!"

We've all done it. As we're headed out the door to dinner, we turn to a friend or our spouse and ask, "Do I look fat in this?" or "Can you tell I've put on a few pounds?"

The person we've put on the spot freezes, stumbles, and says, "Well... I think that dress is flattering."

Isn't it amazing how mixed-up our motives can get? We want honesty from those around us. But we also want reassurances that we don't look as unattractive as we fear. Sometimes we're actually angry at ourselves about how we look, but it's more convenient to feel hurt by another's comments.

If asked, most of us would agree that we want others to be honest with us. But first we must commit to do the same—not to be double-minded in our questions or set traps we know others will step in.

Making this change invites some healthy introspection: *What am I really after when I ask this person this question? How have mixed motives on my part made it difficult for others to encourage or compliment me?* It might help to seek genuine feedback on this issue from those who support you. Assure them that you want to ask only honest questions, and promise them you'll do your best to receive their honest answers like a kiss!

Food for Thought
An honest answer requires an honest question.

A Prayer for Power

Dear God,
thank You for all those people who deeply love me
and who genuinely support my efforts
to improve my appearance and well-being.
Thank You for family members
who really don't mean to say the wrong thing at the wrong moment.
Thank You for friends
who offer a compliment when I am inviting their criticism.
Forgive me, Lord, for those times when I have
sabotaged them, used them, rebuffed their praises,
or decided to take offense over a careless word.
With Your help,
I pray that only true and honest motives
will lie behind the questions I ask
and the approval I seek.
I don't want to be double-minded, manipulative,
weak, or selfish in my relationships.
Heal me through and through, Lord,
for You desire truth in the inner parts (Ps. 51:6).
May these words describe my heart.
Amen.

54 | Under the Influence

Do not get drunk on wine, which leads to debauchery. Instead, be filled with the Spirit.

EPHESIANS 5:18

Just as spending time with a bottle of whisky puts you under the influence of alcohol, an hour with Jesus puts you under the influence of the Holy Spirit. While the one may lead to debauchery—another word for indulgence—the other leads to "love, joy, peace, patience, kindness, goodness, faithfulness, gentleness, and self-control" (Gal. 5:22-23)!

You can spot someone under the influence of Jesus. We see a great example of this in Scripture after the apostles Peter and John were brought before the Sanhedrin. "When they saw the courage of Peter and John and realized that they were unschooled, ordinary men, they were astonished, and they took note that these men had been with Jesus" (Acts 4:13).

When you meet people today, will they notice something unusual about you? Will they wonder if you've been spending time with Jesus?

If you need courage and grace, if you want to be influenced by God, *not* your appetites, follow Mother Teresa's advice in *A Gift for God:* "Put yourself completely under the influence of Jesus, so that he may think his thoughts in your mind, do his work through your hands, for you will be all powerful with him to strengthen you."

Food for Thought

Drink of Jesus, and get under the influence of the Holy Spirit.

A Prayer for Power

Dear God,
I have been under the influence of many things—
including food, lust, laziness, selfishness, pride, and greed,
to name a few of the worst.
And I have also been under the influence
of Your Holy Spirit.
How much better it is to be
moved by You, Lord.
How good it is to know
You are at work powerfully inside of me right now,
motivating me toward right choices
and healthy living.
May I drink deeply of all that You are.
I am desperate for Your living water,
which intoxicates me with love, peace, and joy.
How good it is to know that You are receiving—and answering—
my daily prayers of consecration
with great gladness.
Amen.

55 | Fresh Mercies

His mercies never come to an end; they are new every morning.

LAMENTATIONS 3:22-23, NRSV

There's a reason God's mercies are new every morning. As we travel through this life, we fail God, ourselves, and others every day. On our journey toward healthy living, there will be weak days, tired days, days when we take two steps back from the five steps of progress we made the previous week.

As Simon Tugwell writes in *Prayer,* "One day we may have faith to move mountains and find ourselves the next day scarcely able to rise above twiddling our thumbs hoping nothing [bad] is going to happen."

It's easy to imagine with every setback that God is disappointed and disgusted. But He's not. Luis Palau says, "God is not disillusioned with us. He never had any illusions to begin with."

God is interested in our journey much more than our final destination. Whether you are two steps back today or five steps ahead, you are on the road to transformation. And staying on the road with Him is what matters! God's patience never runs out. He won't throw in the towel, even when you do.

So exchange any regret for repentance. Confess your failure, confident that God has just as quickly forgiven it. Get up and dust yourself off. Take God's hand again, and you'll be able to take the next step forward. Today is a brand-new day, full of brand-new mercies.

Food for Thought
For every fresh failure there is a fresher mercy.

A PRAYER FOR POWER

Dear God,
how do You do it?
How do You put up with my endless mistakes and failures?
One day I take great strides;
the next day I plop myself down and refuse to move forward.
So often I am rebellious and stubborn and lazy.
But every day You meet me here,
ready to take my hand,
mercy and forgiveness shining in Your eyes.
Is this the journey You had in mind?
I want to be faithful to this path and its disciplines, Lord.
Help me not to stay stuck or to turn back
because I underestimate Your loving-kindness
Like fresh spring flowers in the first light of morning,
may I delight in Your mercies as I start each day.
May their fragrance of forgiveness reach me,
and may I open my soul to receive them.
Thank You, generous and faithful Lord.
Renew me with new mercies.
Lead me along the way,
one step at a time.
Amen.

56 | Watch the Salt

As soon as they had brought them out, one of them [an angel] said, "Flee for your lives! Don't look back, and don't stop anywhere in the plain!"... But Lot's wife looked back, and she became a pillar of salt.

GENESIS 19:17,26

Have you ever wondered why Lot's wife, against the advice of angels, just *had* to look back? Was she wanting one last nostalgic look, or was she worried about something she'd left behind or maybe angry about her husband's choice?

Whatever her motive, she's become a symbol of the dangers of looking back when we shouldn't, hanging on to the past instead of the future.

And why did God choose to turn this woman into a pillar of salt? During Bible times, salt was valued as a seasoning but also as a preservative for meats since they didn't have refrigeration. Perhaps God was saying, "Fine! If you want the past, I'll preserve it—and you—forever."

Sometimes it's necessary and even healthy to revisit our past. But retrospection, like salt, should be used sparingly. Remember, you're not working to become what you once were—in weight or size or condition—but the best you can be *today.* Ask God to show you those pivotal moments when a past lesson is just the right spice for a present problem or when He is saying, "Don't look back—and don't stop moving forward!"

Food for Thought
Don't preserve the past, but persevere for your future.

A Prayer for Power

Dear God,
I regret a lot of things I've done,
and I regret even more things I never did
but should have.
But I don't want to waste my present
focusing on the past.
What could have been will never be,
and yet, what still can be is wonderful!
Thank You for caring enough about me
to redirect my eyes toward the future,
to speak to me a gentle warning
in those important moments when looking back might not be best.
As I let go of yesterday
and set my sights on the road I'm traveling right now,
I ask for Your guidance.
Lead me where You want me to go.
Create a spirit of integrity within me.
Help me to persevere in all my commitments,
especially those that affect my health.
Don't let me meet a salty end, Lord!
But let me meet You,
follow You,
and take the next step forward.
Amen.

57 | The Full Treatment

[I am] confident of this, that he who began a good work in you will carry it on to completion until the day of Christ Jesus.

PHILIPPIANS 1:6

Once God has begun to live in you, He doesn't ever stop the process of transformation. You are a beautiful work in progress!

But here's the catch: Maybe you only signed up for limited repairs—those that affect your ability to live a healthy life, for example. You want to learn self-control, lose some weight, get fit. Yet God is not content to stop there.

C. S. Lewis writes in *The Joyful Christian,* "Dozens of people go to Him to be cured of some particular sin with which they are ashamed...or which is obviously spoiling daily life (like bad temper or drunkenness). Well, He will cure it all right: but He will not stop there.... He will give you the full treatment."

Have you been saying to God, in essence, "Bleach my teeth so I'll look better, but please ignore any cavities"? How much better to sign up for the full treatment!

Open every door of your heart to Him today. Invite Him to work in every room that needs His attention, even where it feels painful. Remember, He has only your best in mind. "'For I know the plans I have for you,' declares the LORD, 'plans to prosper you and not to harm you, plans to give you hope and a future'" (Jer. 29:11).

Food for Thought
Treat yourself to God's full treatment.

A Prayer for Power

Dear God,
could it be true?
Have I come to You wanting You
to fix the things about my life that bother me
but not worrying about the things that bother You?
May it not be so!
May I seek to be changed by You in every way,
in every corner of my heart.
Search me, show me—
gently, please, Lord.
Where is there a hidden sin gaping
like a cavity in my soul?
Let Your loving touch fall upon it.
I don't want to pick and choose
what we will deal with, Lord.
Even if it is painful for the moment,
I want the good plans—the hope and future—You have for me!
I open myself to Your Holy Spirit right now,
to Your nudgings, to Your conviction.
I surrender to You all that I am
so that You can make me
all that You intend.
Amen.

58 | Veggies with Love

Better a meal of vegetables where there is love than a fattened calf with hatred.

PROVERBS 15:17

Maybe a fattened calf doesn't sound that tasty to you, but in Bible times it was the ultimate feast. Another way of putting Solomon's words might be, "Better to have canned soup at a happy dinner table than lasagna Florentine when everyone's fighting."

Have you ever noticed that when you are having a good time at dinner and people are laughing and talking, you eat less? It's no coincidence. Enjoying meals in an environment that is uplifting not only makes food less important, but it also helps your digestion.

Mary, a mother of four young kids, realized that the stress, havoc, and squabbling at mealtimes was making her focus on her food for distraction and comfort, causing her to eat too much. Now, by taking time to set a nice table, light candles, say grace—even at lunchtime—the kids sense that this is a special time to enjoy one another rather than just a chance to gobble food while continuing their play. And Mary is more aware of what she's eating and is able to slow down and enjoy each bite.

Food for Thought
Food tastes best with love.

A PRAYER FOR POWER

Dear God,
please help me to make getting along at mealtimes
as important as getting full!
Your Word teaches that veggies with love is a feast.
I don't want to spoil a meal
by eating on the run,
squabbling at the table,
or watching TV while I'm wolfing down
Your gracious provision.
Help me to enjoy what You provide
by serving it always in an atmosphere
of love and peace.
Because of Your power at work in me,
I will make harmony and smiles
and patience and forgiveness
and good listening and good humor
the most important nourishment at my table.
Amen.

59 | Get a Life!

Is not life more important than food?

MATTHEW 6:25

These few words of Scripture have to do with our needless worrying about food and clothing. But they also say something important to the dieter: Your life should not be about food. Your life should be about *life!*

Studies show that women who have few hobbies and interests tend to struggle with their weight more than women who have full lives. It makes sense. The more time we have on our hands, the more bored we become…and the more tempting the refrigerator. Pretty soon our whole life shrinks down to a war against that very thing—food—which God intended to give us energy to live full, productive lives.

Jennifer, a mother of two small children, says, "I kept trying so many diets. My life revolved around them. But finally God showed me that my problem was not dieting, but getting my focus off of the dieting problem and on *living*. I took up two new hobbies I could enjoy with my daughters: hiking and painting with watercolors. I began to try to make more friends, to stay busy. And guess what? When dieting ceased to be my main hobby, I lost the weight."

How about you? If your tummy seems never to be full, consider whether your life is full enough. Invite God to "mess" with your life. And listen for any change of plans He might have in mind for how you spend your time.

Food for Thought
Fill your life with—life!

128

A Prayer for Power

Dear God,
fill my life with the stuff of life.
Help me to empty out any preoccupations or habits
that divert my attention and distract me
from what really matters.
You made this world so full of good things
to see, to experience, to participate in!
I don't want to miss a moment that was meant for me.
I don't want to miss meeting a person I was destined to know.
I give You permission, Lord,
to tamper with, alter—to totally transform my life
Go ahead. Open doors. Call me up.
Show me where to go, what to do,
and I will follow You
anywhere.
Amen.

60 | Husbands and Other Obstacles

Two are better than one.... If one falls down, his friend can help him up.

ECCLESIASTES 4:9-10

It's hard to underestimate the role that our husbands or family members play in encouraging our healthy choices. Some women, like Belinda—forty and married for twenty years—say they could never have achieved their eating and lifestyle goals without their husbands' help.

Others, like Marsha, married for three years, count their husbands among their greatest obstacles. "He doesn't mean to make me stumble. But he's always trying to get me to eat something I'm not supposed to. He thinks by encouraging me to indulge he's saying, 'Go ahead—I love you just the way you are!' And sometimes, I admit, I take advantage of his 'permission.'"

So how do you get your husband or family to support you rather than trip you up? Experts say that the keys are to establish ground rules clearly and to explain your reasons. For example, say, "Please don't encourage me to reward myself with food. When you do, it reinforces my habit of using food the wrong way."

Evaluate when and how you feel encouraged or discouraged by the significant people in your life, and tell them. Confide in them your "triggers" or weak areas, and ask for their help. Once they realize you are serious about your goals, most people close to you will get serious about encouraging you.

Food for Thought
Help your family and friends to help you.

A Prayer for Power

Dear God,
how can I thank You enough
for the people who love me?
I know that no one in my family or group of close friends
wants anything but the best for me.
But sometimes when I need their help,
they fail me.
They are human, Lord.
And sometimes, I know that I am
hard to help!
Give me wisdom in how I ask for the support I need
Give my family and friends wisdom
to know the best way to provide it.
May I never neglect the powerful strength
that is available to me through others.
Two are better than one, indeed!
Amen.

61 | Nothing Is Impossible

What are those feeble Jews doing? Will they restore their wall? Will they offer sacrifices? Will they finish in a day? Can they bring the stones back to life from those heaps of rubble—burned as they are?

NEHEMIAH 4:2

Do you ever feel like the Jews must have felt after they returned from Babylon and were surrounded by broken walls and heaps of rubble—overwhelmed, ashamed, hopeless?

When your efforts to rebuild your life and body into something beautiful feel futile, remember that you do not labor alone. When you are discouraged and defeated, God, for whom all things are possible, is able to empower you with the courage of Nehemiah, who determined to rebuild the walls of Jerusalem (Neh. 2:17).

Claim His promises of physical and spiritual renewal for yourself and for any others you know who could say with the Israelites, "All that we treasured lies in ruins" (Isa. 64:11).

Here are some reassurances for today:

- In time God will bestow on you a crown of beauty instead of these ashes (Isa. 61:3).
- He is merciful toward you, and He promises new things in the midst of old (Isa. 42:9).
- He will heal your deepest hurts (Jer. 17:14).
- He will enable you to be a "Repairer of Broken Walls" (Isa. 58:12).

Food for Thought
God specializes in the impossible.

A Prayer for Power

Dear God,
I know that with You
nothing is impossible.
But sometimes my whole life
feels like an impossible project.
Old wounds, crumbled dreams, and missed opportunities
litter the path to here.
Some of me lies in ruins.
Some things feel as if they can't ever be fixed.
But I know You are a relentless redeemer, Lord.
You are even now kneeling in the rubble of my life,
looking for ways to turn bad to good,
to restore what is broken,
to renew what is worn out,
to revive what is dying or dead.
Today I invite You,
builder of temples, healer of hearts,
to have Your way in repairing what is broken in me
until that day when I leave this damaged home
and I become perfect in Yours.
Amen.

62 | Source of Strength

My heart pounds, my strength fails me; even the light has gone from my eyes....
I wait for you, O LORD; you will answer, O Lord my God.

PSALM 38:10,15

"O Lord, help us to never think that we can stand by ourselves and not need you." John Donne's prayer seems like a simple idea at first glance. But how difficult this truth is to actually live out!

Our first impulse when faced with a difficult challenge is to try harder, to muster our own will power, to call on our own strength. We imagine we don't need God because everything appears to be going along well enough without Him.

Then eventually, once we've pushed too hard and it feels as if we've got nothing left, we collapse into God's arms.

How much better simply to begin there?

Today invite God to come close and wrap you in His strong and tender arms. He delights in being the One to hold you up.

Food for Thought
God will give me strength
when I'm willing to give Him my weakness.

A Prayer for Power

Dear God,
when my strength is gone,
be my strength for me.
When I get to the end of my rope,
meet me there with Your power and Your amazing grace.
When I fall because I have pridefully trusted
in my own wisdom or strength,
help me reach out in trust to You again.
Thank You for the assurance
that whatever my day brings
or whatever You put before me,
You'll give me the strength I need.
Amen.

63 | Excuses, Excuses

The man said, "The woman you put here with me—she gave me some fruit from the tree, and I ate it."

GENESIS 3:12

Since the dawn of time, human beings have been making excuses or blaming others for eating what they shouldn't.

In her book *When Food Is Love,* Geneen Roth says, "When compulsive eaters tell me...more or less, that their eating is someone else's fault, I answer that there are many things in life beyond our control, but our eating is not one of them; it is, however, a perfect reflection of what we believe about responsibility, autonomy, and blame."

If you're caught up in a cycle of excuses or blame shifting—"It was the only thing in the fridge" or "My husband wants fattening meals"—then you're not taking responsibility for your choices. And by hiding from the truth that you alone are responsible for eating what you shouldn't, you miss out on the opportunity for empowering personal change.

Think about it. Even when we try to hide behind excuses and fig leaves, our soul lies naked before God. He sees every motive, every excuse, every little manipulation. If you try to cover up your destructive behaviors, your shame will only drive you further into failure.

It's time to come out of hiding! Unlike Adam and Eve, you haven't been banished from God's garden. He continues to call for you, and when you step out into the light of truth, He is ready to help you face the facts about yourself and give you power to make better choices.

Food for Thought
There's no excuse for excuses.

A Prayer for Power

Dear God,
I know it's true that too often I make excuses
rather than take responsibility for my choices.
And by doing so,
I don't receive the help and the love You long
to lavish on me.
I don't want to hide behind fig leaves, Lord.
You see me as I am.
Right now every corner of my soul lies naked before You.
Help me to remember, Lord, that when
I come to You honestly with my failures
and ask for grace,
You will not condemn me.
Forgive me for making excuses
when I should be making positive changes.
Deliver me from the convenient lies I tell myself
and from the deceptions that keep me stuck in failure and shame.
Today, with Your help, I will not make excuses,
but I will make the truth about me and You
my only defense.
Amen.

64 | Me? Special?

For you created my inmost being; you knit me together in my mother's womb....
How precious to me are your thoughts, O God! How vast is the sum of them!

PSALM 139:13,17

How special do you feel?

That may seem like a silly question. But for most us who don't see Cindy Crawford or Naomi Campbell or even the average TV weathercaster when we look in the mirror, it's an important one.

Your answer probably indicates that too often you feel about as special as your mother's kitchen wallpaper. At times you curse your metabolism, lament your genes, doubt your IQ, and despise your body. "Special?" you mumble as you try to sneak past that dreadful full-length mirror. "How could somebody special have a middle like that?"

Today God wants to remind you of this: He made you on purpose—knitted you together with divine genius—as an expression of His joy. Imagine that! Instead of lamenting all you are not, focus your thoughts today on who you *are*. You are God's unique creation. You have a particular temperament and body type. What works for Cindy or Naomi—or your best friend, Marge—might or might not work for you. That goes for your dieting disciplines as well as every other area of your life.

Today walk out into your world, talk about yourself, and carry yourself as if you are God's special creation, precious in His eyes. Because that is what you are!

Food for Thought
The biggest mistake is to imagine God made a mistake
when He made you.

A Prayer for Power

Creator God,
how priceless is Your every thought about me!
Right now I offer up to You all that I am,
could be,
hope to be,
and will be.
What do You have in mind for my life?
How can I express Your creation miracle in me today?
I will listen all day for Your voice.
I will sing Your praises.
And I will celebrate and share the miracle of You
in me.
Amen.

65 | The Secret of Contentment

I know what it is to be in need, and I know what it is to have plenty. I have learned the secret of being content in any and every situation, whether well fed or hungry, whether living in plenty or in want. I can do everything through him who gives me strength.

PHILIPPIANS 4:12-13

Most of us won't be faced with the dire trials the apostle Paul endured, yet choosing to be content is one of the hardest things to do in life, isn't it? There's always some circumstance or person we wish were different. Paul understood just how difficult being content can be, which is why this topic spurred his famous declaration, "I can do everything through him who gives me strength!"

One of the greatest enemies of contentment just might be the television. After a few hours of viewing "ideal" images, we can come away thinking, *Wow, my husband isn't romantic. My house needs an overhaul. And I am fat and ugly!* As Sheri Rose Shepherd puts it in *7 Ways to Build a Better You,* "If you're watching soap operas all day and your husband comes home, and he doesn't make you feel bold and beautiful and young and restless, you're going to want to put him in the General Hospital."

Today hear God inviting you to turn away from those things that breed discontent. Turn instead toward His personal presence and provision. He wants to give you riches that won't rust, a love for others that endures, and peace that passes understanding.

Food for Thought
Never be content to be discontent.

A Prayer for Power

Dear God,
thank You for being my everything!
Thank You for caring about all
the small struggles I face,
the hollow feelings in my heart,
the way I seek solace.
Thank You for being here now,
ever available, ever capable
of granting me contentment.
Today I ask for the grace and the will
to choose You over any other source
of peace and joy.
Like a baby resting peacefully and contentedly in its mother's arms,
I choose to rest in You.
By Your power at work in me,
I forsake the grumblings of my greedy, anxious nature,
and I embrace gratitude and humility.
I can do this—
I can do all things!—
through Christ who strengthens me.
Amen.

66 | A Spiritual Makeover

Your beauty should not come from outward adornment, such as braided hair and the wearing of gold jewelry and fine clothes. Instead, it should be that of your inner self, the unfading beauty of a gentle and quiet spirit, which is of great worth in God's sight.

1 PETER 3:3-4

Notice here that the apostle Peter isn't saying you *shouldn't* be physically beautiful. He's not condemning caring for your hair or wearing jewelry or nice clothing. But he is saying that real beauty comes from your spirit.

Peter is also not describing a personality, but a spirituality. The word "gentle" here means "restrained power." The woman with a gentle and quiet spirit is strong but under control. She may be funny, boisterous, and even authoritative. But you can tell that she is in submission to Christ, and you get the sense that her heart has received as much attention as her makeup.

Most of us have a beauty regimen. Some of us take an hour in front of the mirror. Others of us slap on our makeup on the way to work. But what kind of *inner* beauty regimen do we have? Are we stepping out today with all the right outer adornment but a sour spirit?

Here's an idea: Develop a daily spiritual regimen, and paste a reminder on your mirror. Try five minutes of quiet and listening, five minutes of Bible reading, and five minutes of prayer. Just as you check your makeup and clothing before running out the door, check your spirit. Is there a smudge of pride to wipe away? Did you forget to put on forgiveness? Regular time in front of a spiritual mirror is the key to lasting loveliness.

Food for Thought
Beauty is an inside job.

A Prayer for Power

Dear God,
how do I look this morning?
I mean, on the inside.
I want to be beautiful there for You, Lord.
Teach me to take the time I need
to accomplish this.
Show me what it truly means
to have a gentle and quiet spirit.
Those aren't the words that most people
would use to describe me.
But now and then I catch a glimpse;
I see what I could be:
lovely within,
calm,
at peace,
confident in You.
That is what I want, Lord!
Can You do it? Can You give me a makeover?
I surrender my soul, with all its blemishes and flaws.
Have Your way within me today, Lord.
Make me look like You.
Amen.

67 | Grow Old Along with Me

Charm is deceptive, and beauty is fleeting.

PROVERBS 31:30

Few words ring more true to millions of woman than "beauty is fleeting."

But is it really? The proverb is actually referring just to physical beauty. It goes on to say, "But a woman who fears the LORD is to be praised."

Having both inner and outer beauty is best, we all agree. Yet, the effects of aging on our physical body are impossible to stop. Part of nature's plan is for wrinkles to appear, for skin to lose some elasticity, for hair to gray. So is it wrong to dye our hair, use wrinkle cream, and do all we can to hide our aging?

That depends on our motives. In her book *Love to Eat, Hate to Eat,* Elyse Fitzpatrick asks, "Could it be that this worship of youth and beauty is a welcome deception as [we] seek to forestall the inevitable for as long as possible, fooling [our]selves into believing that [we] are immortal?"

Our concern for fitness should never end. And there's no reason we should care less about outward beauty as we age. But unlike those who don't love God, we don't have to *fear* aging—or death. And we shouldn't be reinforcing a standard of beauty that isn't God's.

It takes courage to age beautifully. It takes grace to accept laugh lines. Today let every wrinkle remind you that a new, heavenly body awaits you! And the one you have right now deserves nurturing. Above all, respond to God with awe, reverence, and surrender. The best kind of praise begins there.

Food for Thought
Grow old with grace and beauty.

A Prayer for Power

Dear God,
You know that though my body fails,
my face wrinkles,
and my strength leaves me,
on the inside I still feel like a young girl!
Help me not to fret about these outward changes.
Thank You that though outwardly I am wasting away,
inwardly I am being renewed by Your Spirit
day by day (2 Cor. 4:16).
That means my soul is growing more lovely by the minute!
Let me take care to send the right messages about aging
to those around me.
May my comments bring You glory.
May they reflect the hope and affirmation
that every woman can find in You.
May more and more women know
that You love every wrinkle,
every age spot, every new gray hair they find.
Today I choose to celebrate what a wondrous miracle You made
when You made me.
I will welcome the future
with a smile.
Amen.

68 | Just Say No to Perfectionism

Not that I have already obtained all this, or have already been made perfect,
but I press on to take hold of that for which Christ Jesus took hold of me.

PHILIPPIANS 3:12

Have you ever been accused of being a perfectionist? Most of the time we use that word to refer to someone who can't tolerate anything less than perfection from herself or others. Synonyms include "hypercritical," "severe," "demanding," and "fussy."

Jesus wants us to be a perfectionist in another sense. "Be perfect...," He told His disciples, "as your heavenly Father is perfect" (Matt. 5:48). The Greek for the word "perfect" here means "complete" or "mature." Jesus clearly was not saying, "Be perfect on your own." If we could, He would not have had to die for us. Instead, He is saying, "Since you're God's children, strive to be like Him."

We do have a part to play in the pursuit of perfection. The apostle Paul exerted himself and "pressed on," but notice it was not to accomplish his *own* goals. He was trying to attain the same goals Christ had in mind for him when He saved or "took hold" of him.

Today just say no to the prison of perfectionism. Refuse to be critical of others or unforgiving toward yourself. Instead, celebrate your freedom to be whole and mature. Aim to cooperate with God and to share His goals for you. Strive for His kind of perfection, always mindful that Jesus alone is the *perfecter* of your faith (Heb. 12:2). It's another one of God's wonderful paradoxes! To become perfect or "complete" is to be wholly aware that you are perfectly incomplete without Christ.

Food for Thought
Strive to be perfected, but don't be a perfectionist.

A Prayer for Power

Dear Lord,
just the word "perfect" sends chills down my spine.
And yet, You ask me to try!
Thank You that I don't have to try
on my own power.
Thank You that I can reach for completeness,
even admire it as a goal,
only because *You* are perfect.
Keep me from sinful pride
and striving for goals that aren't Yours.
Let me not be a perfectionist in the captive sense—
critical, harsh, unwilling to tolerate weakness.
Instead, make me a free, confident woman
who is always wanting to grow,
always asking You, "What is the next step for me to become mature?"
Today this is my prayer:
Please perfect my heart
and my faith
with Your incomparable presence and peace.
Amen.

69 | That Hurts!

No discipline seems pleasant at the time, but painful. Later on, however, it produces a harvest of righteousness and peace for those who have been trained by it.

HEBREWS 12:11

We've all heard the maxim about exercise: no pain, no gain. The same is true of anything we try to accomplish that involves discipline, including dieting. No matter how good we are at finding delicious alternatives, eventually we will have to deny ourselves a food we really, really want. But we do it because there is something else—a healthy body—that we want more. But the process hurts.

"To cultivate the discipline of delayed gratification," writes Sue Monk Kidd in *When the Heart Waits*, "we have to learn one elemental thing, to face pain."

In *Telling Yourself the Truth*, Marie Chapian and William Backus concur: "It's not easy to go without something you desperately want. But most of the time…you'll find that gaining something valuable in your life will depend on being willing to tolerate distress, anxiety, discomfort and discontent.… You *can* deny yourself. You *can* say no to yourself.… You can stand it. You really can."

Are you willing to experience some pain in order to be trained by discipline? If so, God promises that you will reap the rewards: a harvest of peace and righteousness, and a harvest of health and fitness, too.

Food for Thought
God concurs: No pain, no gain.

A Prayer for Power

Dear Lord,
does it have to hurt?
You know that I don't like pain,
and I hate to deny myself what I want
when I want it.
But I do want the larger goal I'm reaching for.
Teach me discipline, Lord.
Let it train me and change me.
Thank You for Your promise that
the pain of discipline only lasts for a while.
With Your support, I can endure it.
I will not be surprised or sidetracked by it;
instead, I will expect it,
and I will run to You for comfort and power.
You know better than anyone
what it means to deny yourself, Lord.
When I consider what you endured for me,
I feel silly for even mentioning my struggles.
Make me more you like You, God.
May I be ever willing to do Your will,
to deny my fleshly appetites and sinful nature,
in order that I might please You alone
and bring You glory.
Amen.

70 | Hungry for Goodness

Blessed are those who hunger and thirst for righteousness,
for they will be filled.

MATTHEW 5:6

Aside from our physical hungers, we all hunger for many things: for love, acceptance, success at work, achieving our goal of healthy living. We spend a lot of time and energy trying to feed these natural hungers. But Jesus might ask us: How strong is your appetite for righteousness?

Do we want to grow in purity as much as we want to become fit?

Do we want to mature in selfless devotion to others as much as we want to receive their compliments for our appearance?

Unlike our stomach hunger, which automatically signals full or empty, depending on how much food the stomach contains, the way Jesus talks about hunger makes it clear it's something we can choose. We can *decide* to be hungry for righteousness. And here's the good news: All we have to do is want it! Then Jesus promises that we *will* be satisfied. He will give us *His* righteousness and fill us with His bread of life.

Food for Thought
It is good to be hungry for goodness.

A Prayer for Power

Dear God,
I never thought I'd pray to be hungry,
but today I ask that You would give me
a gnawing, driving spiritual hunger
for You and Your righteousness.
I want to thirst for Your presence
and to crave to do what is right.
Thank You for Your promise
that if I hunger to live in a way that honors You,
I will be satisfied.
Let me feel *this* deep longing, then,
more than any other today.
And let me notice and praise You
when I am filled to overflowing.
Amen.

71 | The Diet Police

The pleasantness of one's friend springs from his earnest counsel.

PROVERBS 27:9

A friend's earnest counsel is indeed a pleasant thing. But how *un*pleasant that same friend's counsel can be if she's become your diet cop. Diet cops are people you've drafted, consciously or not, to police you, baby-sit your plate, and "tsk tsk" at appropriate moments. Unlike the diet buddies you count on for support and prayer, you count on these people to make you feel guilty.

Sound crazy? Here's an example: When Debi's husband began, at her request, to ask what she'd eaten during the day, stop her from ordering french fries, and monitor her intake at parties, guess what happened? She began to resent his remarks, sneak food, and binge when she was angry with him. Unwittingly she'd transferred her conflict with food into the center of her marriage.

How can you tell if you've turned someone into a diet cop? Consider your response to his or her "helps." Listen to the tenor of the relationship. Is it suffering from inappropriate role playing? Marta admits, "I enlisted my thin best friend to police me so that she'd see how hard this really is. She ended up preferring lunch with other friends."

If the counsel you're soliciting is not "earnest counsel," then make some changes. Gently and honestly discuss appropriate roles for your friends and family in your dieting efforts. Make it a goal never to put your dieting ahead of any relationship. And always keep loved ones in a position that you and they find pleasant.

Food for Thought
Retire your diet police.

A Prayer for Power

Dear God,
do I have any diet cops in my life?
Show me if I do.
I don't want to harm or abuse
any of the people who love me and try to help me.
I know that I have put others in awkward positions before.
Forgive me.
Help me to enlist the kind of honest, healing,
and appropriate support You know I need.
Send the right people,
the right encouragements,
the right promptings into my life.
Make me open to counsel,
earnest in my efforts to grow and change.
Bless the people in my life and in my family
with the grace and wisdom to know how to truly help me.
Search my heart today,
and show me if there is any person
with whom I need to make changes.
Then show me how to make them gracefully.
Amen.

72 | Give It Up

But when the kindness and love of God our Savior appeared, he saved us, not because of righteous things we had done, but because of his mercy.

TITUS 3:4-5

If there's one thing the apostles emphasized, it was that you can't earn salvation by anything you do. You can't become worthy of God's love or deserving of His forgiveness. You can't become more qualified to sit at God's banquet table in heaven by successfully sticking to your dieting program. If you're trying, give it up!

It slips in, this evil little lie, that we can add to what God has already done. That's partly because the truth contradicts many other experiences we've had. We felt our parents' approval when we were *good.* We studied hard to earn an A. We worked extra hours to qualify for a promotion or a pay raise. Good performance equals reward. Period.

God's approach to relationship with us is so radically, dramatically different that we can hardly take it in. His is not just a sliding scale—it's the removal of the scale altogether! His love is a gift. Free. His affection for us is unbounded. His forgiveness can't be exhausted. His willingness to die for us didn't happen just once but is a constant, ongoing reality.

Lay aside any notion that if you "do well" today, God will love you more. Or that if you fail, He will love you less. His love for you is already complete. Let it overflow into the way you live, the way you love others, and the way you approach your commitments today.

Food for Thought
You don't need to earn God's love.

A Prayer for Power

Dear God,
I am so glad that there's nothing I can do
to make You love me more.
But sometimes I live as though I wish there were.
I imagine wrongly that if I perform well for You
or if I am good all day long,
You will not only be pleased,
but You will also love and accept me more.
I do want to please You, God,
but never let me forget that it is
only by grace, only by gift,
that I am saved from sin,
from myself, from my mistakes.
I can't earn Your love by jumping through hoops of my own making.
Forgive me for trying!
Today give me the grace to take it in—
Your love freely given,
Your affection lavished without restraint,
Your ongoing approval of me,
because of what Jesus did on my behalf.
Amen.

73 | Crash Prevention

The heart is deceitful above all things and beyond cure.

JEREMIAH 17:9

Everyone who embarks on an exercise or weight-loss program will eventually experience setbacks. But how do you keep these small setbacks from escalating into a complete relapse, a return to your old ways?

Because the heart is unbelievably deceitful, one key to crash prevention is to know your own tricks. In *Gentle Eating,* authors Stephen Arterburn, Mary Ehemann, and Vivian Lamphear explain: "Relapse has a predictable pattern that can be broken before it goes too far. First, there is *complacency.* You stop doing all the things that you know are helpful and healthy. Second, there is *confusion.* You wonder if your problem was really as bad as you thought. You convince yourself you have a new outlook that will allow you to handle any situation. Third, you *compromise.* You set yourself in too many high-risk situations to resist. Once you reach that stage it is only a matter of time before the fourth stage, *catastrophe,* hits and you lose control."

Memorize those four *C* words, and keep them in mind as red flags. If you find yourself in one of these stages right now, don't despair. You can turn back—*completely*—with a simple confession and change of course.

Though Jeremiah despaired that there was no cure for the heart's deceitful state, he knew there was hope and help for daily living. Make his declaration your own today: "Heal me, O LORD, and I will be healed; save me and I will be saved, for you are the one I praise" (Jer. 17:14).

Food for Thought
Recognize relapse; reach for rescue.

A Prayer for Power

Dear God,
I am a sneaky creature, aren't I?
Even when I am confident,
moving ahead full throttle toward my goals,
I am vulnerable to my own deceptions.
Teach me how to get smart, God.
Make me aware of those subtle, small moves
that gradually put me off course
and pull my heart away from Yours.
There is no cure for me
other than reaching for the truth
and Your healing touch.
My course is always headed for a crash
without You to direct and protect me.
Thank You that I am not left to make these changes alone.
Thank You that I can count on the nudging of Your Holy Spirit.
Take this heart of mine and make it new, Lord.
Cleanse me, and I will be clean.
Love me, and I will be whole.
Live in my heart, and I will be true.
Heal me, and I will be healed.
Amen.

74 | Ode to Joy

Finally, my brothers, rejoice in the Lord! It is no trouble for me to write the same things to you again.... Rejoice in the Lord always. I will say it again: Rejoice!

PHILIPPIANS 3:1; 4:4

The book of Philippians has been called Paul's ode to joy. Even though the apostle wrote from prison, he repeatedly expressed his own joy and urged his fellow Christians to rejoice, no matter their circumstances.

Paul knew what many people today miss: There's power in joy, *and we can choose it.* Unlike happiness, which is determined by mood or circumstances, the rush of joy can be experienced even in painful, dark times.

Bob Greene, famous for helping Oprah Winfrey lose a lot of weight some years back, believes that "living in the present" is a key to joy, and joy is a key to fitness success. He writes in *Make the Connection:* "I noticed that all the people I worked with were preoccupied with either the past or the future. They never seemed to experience the present. Looking back, I realize that most of these people were never joyful. The two concepts are related. It is much easier to experience true joy when you learn to live 'in the moment.'"

When was the last time you experienced an outpouring of true, soul-deep joy? Especially when you are struggling or discouraged, take time to sit quietly, experience the present, and *choose* joy. Then proclaim with the psalmist: "When I said, 'My foot is slipping,' your love, O LORD, supported me. When anxiety was great within me, your consolation brought joy to my soul" (Ps. 94:18-19).

Food for Thought
Joy is available to you today.

A Prayer for Power

Dear God,
just as You are worthy of my worship,
I know that You are worthy of my rejoicing in You.
But so often I choose to be controlled instead by my circumstances.
On bad days I'm crabby because I feel I have a right to be.
On good days I'm sunny because things are going well.
But that is living according to my emotions,
not living according to the power of Your Spirit.
Show me how to rejoice today,
right now, right here,
in this very moment.
Thank You for making Your joy available to me!
I know that it was for this joy
You endured the shame of the cross.
Let me not miss it.
May I declare with the psalmist,
today and every day,
"This is the day the LORD has made;
I will rejoice and be glad in it" (from Ps. 118:24)!
Amen.

75 | A Gentle Approach

The LORD said, "Go out and stand on the mountain...for the LORD is about to pass by." Then a great and powerful wind tore the mountains apart and shattered the rocks before the LORD, but the LORD was not in the wind. After the wind there was an earthquake, but the LORD was not in the earthquake. After the earthquake came a fire, but the LORD was not in the fire. And after the fire came a gentle whisper. When Elijah heard it, he pulled his cloak over his face and went out and stood at the mouth of the cave.

1 KINGS 19:11-13

Like Elijah, so often we expect God's approach to be harsh, violent, fiery. Instead, He often passes by with a gentle whisper. Hundreds of years after Elijah's experience, Jesus described himself as "gentle and humble in heart" (Matt. 11:29). And Paul preached, "Let your gentleness be evident to all" (Phil. 4:5).

It's not easy to receive God's gentle touch, much less be gentle with ourselves. "Few people have been gentle with us, and we follow their lead and beat ourselves up on the inside," write the authors of *Gentle Eating*. "If we can finally be gentle with ourselves...we may find less reason to soothe our wounds with the needed medication of fat-saturated, sugar-soaked food."

Today, as He does every day, God is going to pass by. But don't look for Him to erupt or explode. Don't listen for a harsh reprimand. Instead, listen for His tender whispers of encouragement. In His gentleness is all the wisdom and power you need. And as you receive His gentle touch, you will learn to be more gentle with yourself and others.

Food for Thought
God's approach is a gentle one.

A Prayer for Power

Dear God,
I want to experience Your gentleness today.
I confess that I am often harsh with myself,
berating and accusing,
undoing the gentle work You are about.
Even while You whisper to me,
I drown You out with my own harsh judgments of myself.
I don't want to do that, Lord!
Teach me Your gentleness, Jesus.
Show me today the path of grace.
Let Your gentleness wash my heart clean
of futile and self-defeating approaches to change.
Quiet my spirit as You pass by
so I will hear Your gentle whisper.
Amen.

76 | Unabashed Passion

My dove in the clefts of the rock, in the hiding places on the mountainside,
show me your face, let me hear your voice.

SONG OF SONGS 2:14

Whether we're single or married, most of us want to feel that we're physically attractive to the opposite sex. But if we imagine that in order to be
sexually desired we must attain a *Playboy* standard of beauty, we will feel
ashamed of our bodies and begin to hide our face—and the rest of us.

Marcia, a mother of five, felt that with every pound she gained she
lost an equal amount of her husband's sexual desire for her. "But when
we finally talked," she says, "the truth came out: I had quit believing in
my physical attractiveness and had withdrawn from sex. Phil wanted me
as much as ever. But he wanted a wife who was responsive, sexually interested, and willing to be seen and touched."

For many women one of the most painful aspects of being overweight is the feeling that they are too fat, too dimpled, too rippled to be
sexually attractive. But your body—as it is right now—is worthy of love,
not rejection.

So show your lover your face—and the rest of you as well. (Okay,
maybe dim the lights a little, or try some alluring lingerie.) Let your mate
embrace your body even as you seek to have your body's appearance reflect
love and care. Believe that you are sexually attractive just as you are—and
you will be more attractive than ever.

Food for Thought
The less self-protective you are, the more passionate you become.

A Prayer for Power

Dear God,
how can such a simple thing
as being naked with my spouse
bring on such feelings of shame?
I don't look the way I imagine he wants me to look.
Or does sexual desire blur his vision
of the reality that is my body?
No, You answer. *Love clears his vision.*
Really, Lord?
Help me not to make assumptions
that lead to distance between my spouse and me.
How can I reach out with desire for him
when I am shrinking from his desire for me?
Change me, Lord.
Fill me with unabashed passion for my husband
that I might tear down these self-centered, protective walls,
and welcome intimacy without shame.
May my marriage bed be remade
into the sacred, sexual, and lovely place You intended.
Amen.

77 | Healing Words

Pleasant words are a honeycomb, sweet to the soul and healing to the bones.

PROVERBS 16:24

In her book *You Are Not What You Weigh,* Lisa Bevere tells a story about coming home from school at age fifteen to have her father ask her to turn around to show him her backside.

"You are getting so fat!" he declared. "Look at your bottom—it's huge!"

"I remember going into my room," she writes, "and stripping myself and looking at myself and thinking, 'I'm disgusting! I'm gross! I'm fat!'"

That's the problem with words that wound: We tend to turn them into mantras, letting them shape the way we think and talk about ourselves.

Do you need to retrain your mouth and heart? You know the power of hurtful words, but never underestimate the power of pleasant words, which are "healing to the bones." Neva Coyle and Marie Chapian, authors of *Free to Be Thin,* suggest that you practice saying these truths to yourself in the mirror:

"I am fearfully and wonderfully made."

"I accept myself."

"I accept and bless my body."

"I will eat and care for my health because I am precious."

"I choose not to abuse myself in any way."

"My body was created to be healthy, and I will cooperate with God to make it so."

Food for Thought
Mantras can hurt or heal you.

A Prayer for Power

Dear God,
thank You that Your words bring life and healing.
Thank You that the truth about me
has nothing to do with words that wound or lie.
Please reach inside my memory,
straight into my past,
and muffle every harmful word
that still pierces me.
Help me to resist repeating any hurtful and untrue statements
as the soundtrack to my life.
May my mouth become a tool of truth
that speaks well and truly of myself and others.
May I speak pleasant words
that bring healing to the core of my being
and bless those around me.
By Your grace and power, Lord,
I will declare Your glories
and repeat only words that bring life.
Amen.

78 | The Land of Temptation

I do not understand what I do. For what I want to do I do not do,
but what I hate I do.

ROMANS 7:15

If you are trying to change your habits, grow in self-control, or become more like Christ, welcome to the land of temptation!

It's been said that no one is tempted to sin as much as the person who is trying not to sin. The moment we decide that a certain course is wrong, we have to resist something we didn't before, which brings temptation into the limelight.

So if you're feeling tempted, don't get discouraged or be alarmed. You are actually on the right track!

Hannah Whitall Smith put it this way in *The Christian's Secret of a Happy Life:* "Strong temptations are generally a sign of great grace, rather than of little grace. And the very power of your temptations…may perhaps be one of the strongest proofs that you really are in the land you have been seeking to enter, because they are temptations peculiar to that land."

It's true! The very fact that you struggle against sin means that you are in the right place, a good place. Don't let temptations discourage or defeat you today. Instead, see them as proof that you are making progress in the right direction.

Food for Thought
The land of temptation is a placc of great grace.

A Prayer for Power

Dear God,
You know that I live in a land of temptation,
a land where each day I must
ask for grace and help from You.
Keep me from mistaking these temptations
as a sign of failure or weakness that will lead
inexorably to my defeat.
Remind me that they exist exactly *because*
I am striving for holiness.
Thank You that You are greater
than any temptation or power.
And You live in me!
Thank You for Your mercies,
which are always greater,
always more complete
than I ever imagine.
Let every temptation chase me
into Your arms,
and grant me the vision to grasp again
the unfathomable greatness of Your grace.
Amen.

79 | Shut My Mouth

Do everything without complaining.

PHILIPPIANS 2:14

Easy for Paul to say, right? The apostle never had to eat rice cakes, say no to cherry cobbler, or try on a bathing suit in the cruel light of a dressing room.

It's easy to whine and moan and let the world know how much we are suffering, how deprived we are. But when we complain about our diets or disciplines, not only do we become tiresome to be around, but we also sabotage our efforts. Mary woke up to this reality. "I realized I was always talking about dieting, mostly complaining, in place of actually *doing* it. Finally I decided to treat my eating as a private goal between God and me. I think the more someone grumbles about losing weight, the longer it will take to happen."

Yes, dieting is hard. Yes, we may be disappointed by our failures or worried about our progress. But we *choose* the way we respond to those things that "cause" us discomfort. In *Telling Yourself the Truth,* Marie Chapian and William Backus concur: "*You* make the choice to be happy. You make the choice to think true thoughts about yourself and others.... You face yourself as you are right now, taking responsibility for your thoughts, feelings, and attitudes."

Today make it a point to listen carefully to what comes out of your mouth. Don't fuss and grumble. "But thanks be to God, who always leads us in triumphal procession in Christ and through us spreads everywhere the fragrance of the knowledge of him" (2 Cor. 2:14).

Food for Thought
Whine a lot, weigh a lot.

168

A Prayer for Power

Dear God,
what do I think I will accomplish by whining?
When I complain about my diet,
my weight,
my dismay over my size,
nothing changes...
even though I fool myself into feeling I've addressed the problem.
I don't want to let talk replace action, Lord.
Help me to turn that impulse to discuss my frustrations and failures
into an impulse to act on the truth.
Help me to watch over my mouth today
so that what comes out not only builds up others,
but builds up me as well.
When I'm tempted to complain,
shut my mouth, Lord!
Bring to my mind only those things that are worthy of words
and worthy of You.
Amen.

80 | Your Father's Lap

How great is the love the Father has lavished on us, that we should be called children of God! And that is what we are!

1 JOHN 3:1

Remember the old song "Jesus loves me, this I know"? It's true. Most of us do know that *Jesus* loves us. But God? Isn't He sorta angry all the time?

Because Jesus came to earth as a man, suffered as a man, and died for us, we tend to cling to this part of the Trinity. Jesus is our friend and brother. God is the stern Father who is disapproving and punishing. Given the choice, we'd rather run to Jesus for help with our problems.

If you realize that you tend to avoid "God the Father," it may mean that you have some unresolved issues about or unhealed wounds from your earthly father. Long after we've grown up, our childhood relationship with our father continues to influence how we feel about our sexuality and our femininity, how we relate to men, how we feel about our bodies, and above all how we relate to *Abba,* our heavenly daddy.

If your father was abusive, absent, or emotionally unavailable, consider finding some help to address and heal these hurts. Read helpful books, see a counselor, journal, talk to a trusted friend.

God invites you not just to a throne room to worship Him on high, but onto His lap where He can lavish His love on you.

Food for Thought

God *is* the daddy you always dreamed of.

A Prayer for Power

Dear God,
when I think of You,
when I approach You as my Father in heaven,
I'm not sure I'm seeing You clearly.
And I want to!
Sometimes I feel ashamed, embarrassed even,
to relate to You the way Your Son Jesus did.
I know You are my *Abba*, my "daddy,"
but I need Your help to convince my heart.
I pray for healing in any parts of my soul
where the word "daddy" isn't at home.
I pray that my past would stay where it belongs,
that it might not interfere with my relationship with You now.
You know the way I must go
the work I must do,
to heal my hurts.
Show me how to climb onto Your lap today.
I want to *feel* Your love.
I'm reaching for You.
Please reach for me.
Amen.

81 | A Remedy for Rejection

I have chosen you and have not rejected you.

ISAIAH 41:9

This small sentence is saying two very important things: Not only has God chosen you, picked you out, deemed you lovable and worth dying for, but He also hasn't rejected you. And He never will.

We've all experienced the pain of rejection—by a friend, a parent, an employer perhaps. We know what it is to approach someone, to feel vulnerable, hopeful, and needy, only to be rejected. No one understands this feeling more than Jesus, whose love was scorned and turned away by the very people He came to redeem. "This is the New Testament picture of Jesus," writes Brennan Manning in *Lion and Lamb.* "He is spurned, avoided, treated as a leper, a born loser."

Having experienced the ultimate rejection, Jesus is your ultimate sympathizer and comforter when you experience rejection. He will, again and again, *choose* you. And not because He's obligated to or because you're automatically included in His Father's grand redemption plan for the human race. You *in particular* have been chosen, loved, and pursued by Him!

Whenever you feel that sting of rejection, whenever someone in this world says, "You're not the one I want," hear God say, "I have chosen you!" And let Him apply to your hurt the healing balm of His love.

Food for Thought
Rejection hurts, but being chosen heals.

A Prayer for Power

Dear God,
rejection does hurt.
In fact, it hardly hurts any less today
than it did when I was a little girl,
desperate to be included by friends and praised by teachers.
I always wanted to be picked,
and I still do.
It is so wonderful to remember that You do choose me.
You want me, and You not only love me,
You like me!
When I feel the sting of this world's rejection for whatever reason,
may I find my solace and comfort in You.
You, who suffered the worst and most unwarranted rejection,
understand exactly what it feels like to be disregarded,
tossed aside, insulted, scorned.
Today I want to identify with You in Your suffering (1 Pet. 4:13)
so that, like Paul, I may share in Your glory (Rom. 8:17).
Help me to understand all that this implies, Lord.
And may each rejection I experience here
on behalf of You or directed at me
take me one step further into the healing depths
of Your love.
Amen.

82 | Dearly Beloved

Be imitators of God, therefore, as dearly loved children and live a life of love.

EPHESIANS 5:1-2

When you lose five pounds, do you feel more worthy of love?

In *7 Ways to Build a Better You,* Sheri Rose Shepherd recalls how losing weight affected her thinking. "Everybody said, 'Oh, you look great. You look wonderful....' I thought, *You know what? When I'm thin, I deserve love. When I'm thin, I'm accepted. When I'm fat,...I don't deserve love. When I'm fat, I need to be rejected.*"

Does this kind of thinking sound familiar? Many health experts believe that one reason women pack on excess weight is to create a safe barrier—in essence, to repel intimacy and refuse to receive the love we feel we don't deserve. As a result of our low self-esteem, we rebuff our husband's sincere sexual advances, or we perceive an encouraging comment from a friend as an insult.

The fact is, only when we choose to believe the truth that we are "dearly loved children" can we begin to "live a life of love." Just as we love Christ because He first loved us, it is only by first *receiving* love that we have love to give others. And get this: Love is our most powerful ally in our battle against self-destructive lifestyle habits! The more we allow ourselves to be loved, the less inclined we are toward self-abusing choices.

Today ask God for the courage to believe in the greatest news of all: *I am dearly loved!*

Food for Thought
Don't refuse love; *use* love.

A Prayer for Power

Dear God,
because You say it is true,
I know it is so: *I am dearly beloved!*
I am loved by You through and through,
and I am loved by many other people, too.
I don't want to push them away!
I don't want to think, "I'm not worth loving!"
Give me the courage instead
to receive love with grace and gratitude.
May I always be ready to turn the love I get
into love that I give away.
And may my growing belief in the fact that I'm loved
be one more reason to treat my body with care.
Thank You, God,
that I am Your dearly loved child!
Because this is true,
I can live a life of love—
received and returned.
Amen.

83 | A Dry and Weary Land

O God, you are my God, earnestly I seek you; my soul thirsts for you,
my body longs for you, in a dry and weary land where there is no water.

Psalm 63:1

How would you describe the landscape of your heart today? Is it a dry and weary land? Or are you feeling energized and satisfied?

It's no secret that our emotional state is a strong determiner of how we will respond to challenges and temptations. When we're depressed or frustrated, we want to say, "Oh hogwash! I give up! It's no use!"

No one recorded these feelings more eloquently than David, the psalmist. But during those down, dry days, he still chose to earnestly seek God. He began many of his prayers and songs with an anguished cry for help, a declaration of despair. But as he encountered God, even beating on His chest as it were, David was also able to fall into God's arms. As he reminds himself, "I have seen you in the sanctuary and beheld your power and your glory" (Ps. 63:2). Spiritual truths triumph over emotional woes.

When you are in a dry and weary place, go to God even if it's the last thing you feel like doing. Tell Him your honest feelings (He knows them already). Remember His faithfulness in the past. Then say in faith with David, "Because your love is better than life, my lips will glorify you.… My soul will be satisfied as with the richest of foods, with singing lips my mouth will praise you" (Ps. 63:3,5).

Food for Thought
When you're in a dry place, seek the Water of Life.

A Prayer for Power

Dear God,
why did You make us such emotional creatures?
My moods get me into all kinds of trouble.
Thank You that with You I don't have to pretend
I am feeling something different than I am.
Thank You that I don't have to *feel* victorious or cheerful or optimistic
in order for You to welcome me and give me victory.
Sometimes it's only after I have spent time with You,
railing or crying or confessing my sadness,
that I begin to see the light of hope.
Show me how to live with my emotions
without letting them live my life for me.
Show me how to be honest about my pain
without letting it deceive or overpower me.
I thank You for the gift of moods and emotions,
even though I don't always welcome them.
You wanted us to be truly alive, didn't You?
When I'm in a dry, weary place,
may I continue to remember the truth:
The best place to go is to You.
Here I am, Lord.
Take me in Your arms, and hear me cry.
Amen.

84 | "The Devil Made Me Do It"

Your enemy the devil prowls around like a roaring lion looking for someone to devour.

1 PETER 5:8

The Bible paints a pretty scary picture of the devil. Imagine a huge hungry lion who is out hunting for his next meal. He spots you lingering in front of the refrigerator full of yummy leftovers. Look out! This is an accurate picture of the kind of opportunity Satan enjoys. But although Satan acts like a hungry lion, he doesn't look like one. As Gwen Shamblin puts it in *The Weigh Down Diet,* "You really have to be on your toes to see the hand of Satan. He does not show up at your house in a red suit with a pitchfork.... His tactics are to remain in the background and chip away at us, or have us lose the battles so subtly that we don't even know that we are in a battle—much less losing it—like a boat slowly drifting to the sea."

Before you despair, listen to this promise you can count on: "Submit yourselves, then, to God. Resist the devil, and he will flee from you" (James 4:7).

Isn't it good to know that God is far stronger than His enemy? The devil can't "make" you do a thing. But you can make the devil hightail it whenever you tell him flat out, "I choose to obey God! Get lost!"

Food for Thought
The devil didn't make you do it.

178

A Prayer for Power

Dear God
thank You that I don't need to fear the devil
or any evil power.
You are so much greater and more powerful
than anyone or anything that opposes You!
Thank You, God, that when the devil sees You inside of me,
he becomes like the cowardly lion in *The Wizard of Oz.*
Thank You for promising me that if I resist evil by Your power,
evil will leave me alone.
Each day help me to stay alert to temptation
or any kind of spiritual attack.
Thank You that You are King over all.
I want You to be the Supreme Power in my life each moment.
Amen.

85 | "Do You Want to Get Well?"

One who was there [at the pool called Bethesda] had been an invalid for thirty-eight years. When Jesus saw him lying there and learned that he had been in this condition for a long time, he asked him, "Do you want to get well?" "Sir," the invalid replied, "I have no one to help me into the pool when the water is stirred. While I am trying to get in, someone else goes down ahead of me." Then Jesus said to him, "Get up! Pick up your mat and walk." At once the man was cured; he picked up his mat and walked.

JOHN 5:5-9

This story of healing makes a surprising point: Jesus knew that if this invalid man were to be healed, his whole way of life would change. He'd be expected to make a living, find a new home, and become a productive member of society. Did he truly *want* to be healed if these were the conditions?

Similarly, we can become so used to our "condition" of overeating and yo-yo dieting that it's become a way of life that we may not really want to give up. In her book *When Food Is Love,* Geneen Roth explains why the problem can become more compelling than the cure: "You never have to do anything but absorb yourself in the cycle of losing and gaining weight to feel that you are involved in something exciting,"

Today hear Jesus asking, "Do you want to get well?" And rather than go over all your excuses for why you're still in the state you're in, ponder what you *really* want. Consider the consequences and challenges inherent in the dramatic change you seek. Do you still want to change? Then ask Jesus in faith to answer your prayer.

Food for Thought

Asking for healing is not the same as wanting it.

A Prayer for Power

Dear God,
I truly do want to be healed!
At least I think I do.
Show me if there is any part of me that has become content
with a cycle of striving and failing.
I don't want to sit poolside any longer.
I surrender my excuses—
all the reasons why I can't seem to overcome
certain familiar sins or cycles of defeat.
I am ready,
I am willing.
I want to be whole!
I want my life to be full and exciting because I am living it for You.
Don't let me be seduced by the subtle lie
that life is more meaningful when I am wrapped up
in a war with my appetites.
Deliver me.
Heal me, and I will take up my life,
new, fuller,
and give You all my thanks and praise.
Amen.

86 | A Family Affair

She gets up while it is still dark; she provides food for her family.

PROVERBS 31:15

It may be an ancient proverb, but today it's usually still the woman who feeds her family. And one of the most challenging aspects of trying to eat healthy is getting our family to cooperate—happily.

Brenda, a stay-at-home mom, says, "I feel I have to make separate meals—steak and potatoes for hubby and kids, fish and veggies for me." Peg, who works full-time but is also in charge of shopping, has a family squawking in protest over the sudden absence of chips and cookies in the cupboards. What's the solution?

Ultimately, any lifestyle change will be more likely to succeed if it involves your whole family. And it stands to reason that if God is calling you to honor Him in the way you care for your body, He wants the same for your family.

Some tips for gaining family cooperation: Abandon the word "diet" around them, and adopt the word "healthy." Gradually try to help change the way your entire family thinks about food. Avoid using it as entertainment or a reward. Instead of banishing all snack foods, slowly replace many of them with plenty of delicious but healthy alternatives.

As your family adopts more healthy habits, you'll notice increased energy and fewer mood swings (often induced by excess sugar). And in the end, this will be true of you: "Her children arise and call her blessed; her husband also, and he praises her" (Prov. 31:28).

Food for Thought
Healthy families are happier.

A PRAYER FOR POWER

Dear God,
today I praise You for my family!
When I think about how much I love them,
I regret the times I resent the work it takes
to keep our household intact and food on the table.
Forgive me, and give me a grateful heart, Lord.
With every meal I serve,
may I be conscious about what I am teaching my family about food,
and about You.
I pray for healthy bodies for everyone who lives in this house.
Do truly bless this food to our bodies!
And make us mindful of the needs of others.
Let every grace we pray ring true,
and let every meal we share remind us
to praise You for Your abundance.
Amen.

87 | Naked and Unashamed

At that moment, their eyes were opened, and they suddenly felt shame at their nakedness. So they strung fig leaves together around their hips to cover themselves.

GENESIS 3:7, NLT

It's safe to assume that Eve could have filled out a healthy size fourteen and felt no shame. But after the big bite, all that changed. Suddenly she knew she was naked, and she was mortified.

It's a feeling many of us experience whenever we stand naked in front of a full-length mirror or undress in front of our mate. No one wants to feel shame, and yet some women insist that such feelings can motivate them to change diet or exercise habits.

Susan asks her friends and her husband to tell her that she's fat and invites them to say mean things "she needs to hear." Jennifer admits, "Some mornings when I get out of the shower, I force myself to stand in front of a full-length mirror and take a long, critical look. Usually I'm so disgusted that I don't blow my diet until at least noon."

In the short term, shame "works" to arouse self-disgust and firm resolve. But as you've probably discovered yourself, the bad and guilty feelings gradually give way to despair and then finally to defeat. The truth is, we don't draw spiritual strength from shame but from right assessments about our human failings and humble repentance before a loving God who is ever ready to meet us in our weakness.

Food for Thought
Shame hurts; love heals.

A Prayer for Power

Dear God,
today I pray for the wisdom to understand the difference between
destructive shame, which accomplishes nothing,
and helpful guilt, which moves me to Your throne of grace.
Teach me how to respect the body You have given me
and even to delight in it.
Thank You that when I stand in Your presence,
naked or clothed,
I don't need to feel shame or humiliation.
Thank You for taking all the guilt for my sins upon Yourself!
Now, fill me with Your Spirit of truth,
which doesn't condemn,
but leads me by loving-kindness to do what is right.
Thank You that where Adam and Eve had only fig leaves
to cover their shame,
I am fully clothed in Your Son's robes of righteousness.
By His power at work in me,
today I choose to honor my body
and treat it with loving care.
Amen.

88 | The Failure of Food

But food does not bring us near to God.

1 CORINTHIANS 8:8

When you consider all the ways we misuse food, thinking it can do what it cannot—comfort, entertain, reward us—it makes sense to spend time remembering what food *can't* do.

Food can't fix your marriage. Food can't make you happy. Food can't heal your wounds. Food can't bring you love. Food can't make you a better parent. Food can't bring you near to God. When it comes to all those things in life that really matter, food is a failure!

But everything food fails to deliver, God does. Listen to the psalmist's declarations of God's "benefits": "Praise the LORD, O my soul, and forget not all his benefits—who *forgives all your sins* and *heals all your diseases,* who *redeems your life from the pit* and *crowns you with love and compassion,* who *satisfies your desires with good things* so that *your youth is renewed* like the eagle's" (Ps. 103:2-5, italics mine).

As the apostle Paul said, "'Food for the stomach and the stomach for food'—but God will destroy them both" (1 Cor. 6:13). Food is for the sustenance and nourishment of your body while you're here on earth. But the things that last for eternity and the things that meet your deepest needs and hungers now are found only at God's buffet table. Today don't seek from food what food will always fail to give. Instead, praise God, and feast on His benefits to your soul's delight.

Food for Thought
Where food fails, God delivers.

A Prayer for Power

Dear God,
today I rejoice in the failure of food!
I rejoice in its failure because it reminds me of Your promises,
which never fail.
You have said, "Love never fails" (1 Cor. 13:8).
May love be what I seek, what I rely on, what I give away, Lord.
For I know that even as I give away love,
I am replenished with love.
Help me never to look to food, to people,
to any kind of outward change, including a better body,
for those benefits that only You deliver.
The plans I make for food beyond physical nourishment
will ultimately fail.
The plans I invest in relationship with You
will always succeed.
Today I will seek true success,
and I will celebrate all of Your benefits:
healing, love, compassion, forgiveness, filling, redemption, renewal!
"Praise the LORD, O my soul;
all my inmost being,
praise his holy name" (Ps. 103:1).
Amen.

89 | A Refreshing Idea

He who refreshes others will himself be refreshed.

PROVERBS 11:25

Sometimes when we're focused on changing habits, it's easy to get wrapped up in our own concerns and begin to isolate ourselves from others. As we strive and labor over our bodies and disciplines, we grow lonely, discouraged, weary with our efforts.

God says one way to be refreshed is to refresh others. Today imagine what someone could do or say that would really refresh and energize you. Maybe it's just a phone call of encouragement, or maybe it's a generous favor—an offer to baby-sit your kids and give you the afternoon off. Then ask yourself: Is there someone I could refresh in a similar way?

Jesus declared, "Give, and it will be given to you. A good measure, pressed down, shaken together and running over, will be poured into your lap. For with the measure you use, it will be measured to you" (Luke 6:38). God's principles aren't just great sayings; they work!

To refresh someone else doesn't have to take a lot of time or even cost you much. It's the effort and intent of giving itself that refreshes your spirit. Mother Teresa said in *A Gift for God*, "To show great love for God and our neighbor we need not do great things. It is how much love we put in the doing that makes our offering something beautiful for God."

Food for Thought

Refresh your spirit by refreshing someone else's.

A Prayer for Power

Dear God,
today I need Your refreshing touch
first of all and most of all.
As I come to You for a second wind,
for an encouraging word,
keep me mindful of those around me who could use the same—
and could receive it from me.
Live through me, Lord.
I know that I am only able to refresh others
because of the refreshment You give me.
Keep me from being so wrapped up in my own worries
that I miss the opportunities You bring my way to give.
Prompt me, nudge me.
Remind me of the many sisters who are struggling just as I am.
Who can I refresh today,
even though I need refreshment myself?
Thank You that Your words are life
and Your ways are true
and whenever I operate according to Your will and principles,
You come through!
Jesus, Restorer of my soul,
I praise You and thank You.
Amen.

90 | When Jesus Shows Up

While they were still talking about this, Jesus himself stood among them and said to them, "Peace be with you."

LUKE 24:36

Have you ever noticed how often Jesus shows up when He's least expected —and without making Himself immediately known? It happened that way for those disappointed followers on the road to Emmaus (Luke 24:13-35). Suddenly Jesus was present, just waiting to be recognized.

Sometimes when Jesus shows up, we don't "see" Him, because in reality we're not looking for Him. Maybe Jesus shows up while you're fighting with your husband. Or He makes Himself known just as you're about to embark on an eating binge.

Simon Tugwell writes in *Prayer,* "If we want to keep company with God…that means that we hand over to him the right to choose how and when to present himself to our consciousness. We all like keeping God in a cupboard with the best china and the family silver, to look at when we feel inclined. But the living God chooses his own times, and will come when he is not wanted."

If God makes an unexpected appearance today, will He be recognized? Wanted?

Here's a radical idea: Ask Jesus to become suddenly present *when you need Him most,* instead of when you want Him. Look for Him all day—in the eyes of friends, in the surprise phone call or visit. Whether He comes with gentle correction or a risky invitation, He always comes in love.

Food for Thought
Watch for God all day.

A PRAYER FOR POWER

Dear God,
be suddenly present to me today.
Show up in a way that I can recognize You,
that I can feel Your intimate presence,
Your loving eyes upon me.
I need You near.
I need You right here.
I am looking for You,
and in my spirit, I'm filled with excitement and anticipation.
I have joy because I know that You really do
walk this earth with us even though I can't see You.
You still speak to Your people, even if we don't always hear.
You still visit us in special, inexplicable ways.
You come, Lord, where and when You are wanted
and sometimes where and when You are not.
I invite You, Jesus, to show up today
when I need You most,
not when I feel most prepared.
I invite You to arrive at any moment,
and I pray that when I see You,
I will really recognize You.
Come, Lord Jesus;
I'm waiting.
Amen.

91 | Cheaters Anonymous

Food gained by fraud tastes sweet to a man, but he ends up with a mouth full of gravel.

PROVERBS 20:17

Few of us would consider a small indulgence not included in our healthy eating plan to be fraud. And in one sense, it isn't. Fraud usually implies that we've taken something from someone else by false means. But when we take and eat what we've committed to ourselves not to eat, don't we defraud *ourselves?*

We've all done it. In a moment of rebellion or conscious uncaring we reach for our child's Halloween candy or we sneak a piece of pie when no one's looking. Then comes regret. It sits there in our stomach like gravel, and we wonder, *Why did I go and do that?*

Rest assured, God is not nearly so worried about the calories or fat you consumed as He is about the state of your heart. He knows you will feel angry with yourself, and His goal is not to make you feel worse. But it's worth asking yourself: *If I'm dishonest in small things, aren't I more likely to be dishonest in big things* (Matt. 25:21)?

If you suspect you're a compulsive cheater, consider: Are you outlawing too many favorite foods rather than limiting them? Are you relying on feelings of failure to make you feel like you're making progress?

If you are caught in a negative cycle and want to stop, ask God to help you make a clean start. He's not fed up; He's on your side. He's not an angry teacher with the paddle but your loving Father who wants you to succeed. He's ready to rescue you from self-fraud—the dumbest kind of cheating.

Food for Thought
Cheaters cheat themselves.

192

A Prayer for Power

Dear God,
I don't even like that word "cheat"!
How ridiculous of me to think that I can somehow get ahead
by committing fraud against myself.
Show me if there is a problem in my approach to dieting
that makes cheating seem worthwhile.
If so, I want to change that, Lord.
I want to feel clean and whole and honest through and through.
I don't want to cheat myself or others or You.
Today I pray for a new hunger for integrity in my deepest being.
May I automatically reject the idea of dishonesty in any form,
be it little white lies, secret binges, or false flattery from others.
I want to be reliable and honest with little things
so that You might trust me with the big things.
But I need Your help.
You are "the way and the truth and the life" (John 14:6),
and I'm counting on You.
Amen.

92 | Heavenly Bodies

But our citizenship is in heaven. And we eagerly await a Savior from there, the Lord Jesus Christ, who, by the power that enables him to bring everything under his control, will transform our lowly bodies so that they will be like his glorious body.

PHILIPPIANS 3:20-21

Not to be grim, but although you're exercising, eating tofu, and trimming up today, tomorrow you could be dead. And then what will all your efforts have gained you?

Those of us working to improve our physical bodies are prone to forget that our true home is heaven. We sweat and strive to make our earthly bodies more glorious, rather than eagerly awaiting our new heavenly bodies, which won't wrinkle, sag, or rearrange themselves in unseemly ways as time passes.

There's nothing wrong with putting effort into improving our bodies. But what we invest on them in the way of time, energy, and discipline should never outstrip what we invest in eternity. Paul pointed out to young Timothy: "Physical exercise has some value, but spiritual exercise is much more important, for it promises a reward in both this life and the next" (1 Tim. 4:8, NLT).

As you seek to harness the power and help of Jesus today, don't lose sight of the bigger picture. Eagerly await His return. "Work out" your spirit, and go about your routines mindful that you are only passing through. You are already the citizen of a better place where your "real" body—a glorious and heavenly one—is waiting for you!

Food for Thought
Be heavenly minded for your earthly good.

A Prayer for Power

Dear God,
I'm so glad it's true!
This body of mine that feels
so resistant to change and improvement,
which fails me and fights me,
is on its way out!
It's not my real body but only a temporary home
for my spirit, and Yours, to dwell in.
I'm eager to make this body the best it can be.
But I want to be more eager
for the new body You will clothe me with in heaven.
In light of this reality,
I choose to give as much care and concern
to my spiritual growth and health
as I do to my efforts at physical fitness.
I will fall short, however,
without Your help.
Fill me to overflowing with Your Holy Spirit.
Make me mindful of heaven's approach.
And let me be of earthly good precisely because
I am heavenly minded.
Amen.

93 | Pressure Sensitive

But we have this treasure in jars of clay to show that this all-surpassing power is from God and not from us. We are hard pressed on every side, but not crushed; perplexed, but not in despair; persecuted, but not abandoned; struck down, but not destroyed.

2 CORINTHIANS 4:7-9

Do you sometimes feel as if you're cracking under the pressures of life? The apostle Paul would say, "Great! This is the perfect opportunity to show the world the difference God's all-surpassing power can make."

You see, people don't recognize God at work in a "perfect" woman—one with no scars, no troubles, no struggles. But Christ is revealed in a woman who has scars as a result of divine healing, serenity in spite of trials, and peace in the face of uncertainty.

Today rejoice that your body is God's jar of clay. Because Christ lives in you, no outside pressure can crush you. Because He is your hope, no heartbreak need end in despair. And though you may stumble and fall, no failure can destroy you.

Paul wrote to the Corinthians, "We were under great pressure, far beyond our ability to endure.... But this happened that we might not rely on ourselves but on God, who raises the dead" (2 Cor. 1:8-9).

Stressed? Anxious? Rely on God's all-surpassing power today by living every moment consciously in His presence and claiming His promises when you need help. He will gently shape you into a woman who reflects His beauty.

Food for Thought
God shines through the cracks.

A Prayer for Power

Dear God,
why would I ever want to rely on myself
when You are so ready to empower and help me?
I feel like the clay jar Paul described.
I crack easily, and I know I'm chipped all over.
But because You live inside of me,
because You are my treasure,
I can put my confidence in You
rather than in my physical body.
I'm willing to be weak, Lord,
if it means You will show Yourself great within me.
I'm willing to be perplexed,
if it means Your wisdom gets a chance to prove itself
as the obvious solution.
I want to rely only on You
and experience Your all-surpassing power!
Take and hold this weak vessel
in Your gentle but mighty hands.
Mold me gently but firmly.
Fill these cracks with Your love.
Amen.

94 | A Compassionate Christ

When he saw the crowds, he had compassion on them.

MATTHEW 9:36

In his book *Lion and Lamb,* Brennan Manning writes:

> What the Lord showed me at the Cenacle was this: before I am
> asked to show compassion toward my brothers and sisters in their
> suffering, He asks me to accept His compassion in my own life, to
> be transformed by it, to become caring and compassionate toward
> myself in my own suffering and sinfulness.... When I am most
> unhappy with myself, I am most critical of others. When I am
> most into self-condemnation, I am most judgmental of others.
>
> ...On the way home from the retreat I was riding the ferry
> from town to the West Bank when I saw an extremely fat and
> homely woman in her mid-twenties who had probably never once
> in her life experienced a look of admiration or interest from a man.
> I wanted to become her, to walk in her obesity, and taste her feel-
> ings of rejection. I wanted her to see the look of tenderness Jesus
> gives her simply because she counts for nothing, because she is
> ignored and rejected by people who attach such importance to
> physical beauty. I wanted her to accept the love of Jesus Christ and
> be so filled with joy that all the human neglect and contempt
> could not rob her of her dignity.

Today experience Christ's deeply felt compassion for you. Then pass
it on with joy to someone who may be a victim of neglect and contempt.

Food for Thought
Receive compassion; spread compassion.

A Prayer for Power

Dear God,
how wonderful it is to know
that You not only forgive my sins,
but You feel compassion for me in my failures!
You identify with me,
You hurt when I hurt,
and You long to help.
Over and over again I read in Your Word
that You were "filled with compassion" for people.
You ached for them;
You ached to heal them, lead them, love them.
And when You see me—
wandering, spiritually lost, hungry for something I can't name—
You are filled with compassion for me.
Help me to receive it, Lord.
Help me to empty myself of my own judgment
and to humbly accept Your loving gaze on me
and Your compassionate touch, which reaches into the core of my soul.
Fill me to overflowing with this compassion,
so much so that I feel and express only compassion
toward every person I meet.
Amen.

95 | A Treasure to Hold Close

I have treasured the words of his mouth more than my daily bread.

Job 23:12

Job valued God's words more than the food that nourished him. Given the choice, he'd rather miss dinner than miss out on time in God's Word.

The prophet Jeremiah also considered a word from God his sustenance. "When your words came, I ate them; they were my joy and my heart's delight" (Jer. 15:16). The writer of Psalm 119 was intent on showing that everything he cared about in life centered on God's revealed truths.

Job and Jeremiah understood that God's words aren't ordinary. They are imbued with power—to nourish our soul, to keep us from sin, to give us joy.

One way to treasure God's Word is to memorize it. But since the word "memorize" makes most of us shudder, instead let's call it "meditating." Take one verse a day—perhaps the one you're reading each day in this book—and continue to bring it to mind as you go about your day. Before you know it, you will have memorized it! More important, it will change the way you think about and respond to life.

Keep in mind that there's limited value in rote memorization. The scribes and Pharisees could quote entire books of Scripture but obviously failed to let God's truths penetrate their hearts. Rather than aiming to impress yourself or others with the amount of Scripture you can quote, make your goal to hold God's Word close, to treasure it. Aim to feed on and to put your entire trust in its promise and its power. Then you will experience the spiritual sustenance that is better than food.

Food for Thought

Hold God's Word close to your heart.

A Prayer for Power

(from Psalm 119)
Dear God,
I praise You today for Your Word.
Thank You for speaking to me—and putting it in writing—
in words I can trust.
I seek You with all my heart;
do not let me stray from Your commands (v. 10).
How much I want to stay pure in thought, word, and deed!
Help me to live by Your Word today (v. 9).
So that I won't sin, I'll take Your truths with me
in my memory and in my heart (v. 11).
Open my eyes that I may see wonderful things
in every Bible verse (v. 18).
Keep me from deceitful ways, and be gracious to me
as Your Word promises (v. 29)!
Turn all my desires toward what is true and lasting
and not toward selfish gain (v. 36).
Turn my eyes from worthless things (v. 37).
Take away the disgrace I dread,
for Your laws are good (v. 39)
and Your promises renew my life (v. 50).
Amen.

96 | Looking Outward

Each of you should look not only to your own interests, but also to the interests of others.

PHILIPPIANS 2:4

It could be said that the opposite of overeating is to focus on feeding and fulfilling other people's needs.

The very act of dieting requires us to pay great attention to ourselves, our choices, our weaknesses. But if we're not careful, self-care can become self-obsession. We develop an oversensitivity to our hungers and appetites and compulsions. This is why the dieter who struggles most is often the one who is most focused on her quest.

What if we were to see our extra weight not so much as evidence of a weak will, but as evidence that we have paid *too* much attention to ourselves? The wrong kind of attention.

Mother Teresa, the epitome of selflessness, wrote in *Heart of Joy:*

> Jesus' words, "Love each other as I have loved you," should not only be a light for us but also a flame to burn away our selfishness.… Let us be like a genuine and fruitful branch of the vine, which is Christ, accepting him in our lives the way he gives himself to us: as truth, which must be spoken; as life, which must be lived; as light, which must shine out; as love, which must be loved; as a way, which must be trodden; as joy, which must be communicated; as peace, which must be radiated; as sacrifice, which must be offered in our families, to our closest neighbors and to those who live far away.

Food for Thought
Don't forget to forget yourself.

A Prayer for Power

Dear God,
I'm willing to look at this.
Are my eyes mostly on me?
Are my thoughts all day long about
how I can get what I need,
what I want?
Even the good things I seek—
to live healthy, to eat wisely—
can be driven by my desire to improve myself,
for myself's sake!
It's boggling, Lord.
Help me, change me, teach me.
I want to look outward more.
I want to see and care about and notice other people,
to feel their needs as if they were my own.
This is such a radical idea.
So different, I confess,
so opposite from my natural tendencies.
But You can change me, Lord,
because You live in me.
Thank You.
Amen.

97 | On the Verge of a Breakthrough

Now there was a man of the Pharisees named Nicodemus, a member of the Jewish ruling council. He came to Jesus at night and said, "Rabbi, we know you are a teacher who has come from God. For no one could perform the miraculous signs you are doing if God were not with him." In reply Jesus declared, "I tell you the truth, no one can see the kingdom of God unless he is born again."

JOHN 3:1-3

Nicodemus came to Jesus for answers to spiritual questions he didn't even know he had. At first Jesus' words confused him. "'How can a man be born when he is old?' Nicodemus asked. 'Surely he cannot enter a second time into his mother's womb to be born!'" (John 3:4).

What Jesus was saying to Nicodemus is that we achieve spiritual regeneration from the inside out, not the outside in. Laws and self-will are futile. "Flesh gives birth to flesh, but the Spirit gives birth to spirit" (John 3:6).

Sometimes it is when we are on the verge of a breakthrough, as Nicodemus was, that nothing makes sense. *Why can't I change? Why do I keep stumbling into the same stupid mistakes?*

We come to Jesus by night with doubts in hand, driven by hope. But rather than offering us a new list of shoulds, Jesus says, "You can't change by following rules, no matter how hard you try! Come to me, begin again, like a newborn baby with nothing to offer. Let go of your own efforts, and I will change you by my Spirit."

Food for Thought

Breakthroughs are spiritual miracles.

A Prayer for Power

Dear God,
thank You that the answer to my sin and my failures
is not a list of rules or a try-a-lot-harder church program.
No—the real answer is a spiritual miracle!
You really do create something brand-new in me!
I want to continue to experience the spiritual regeneration
that You alone can give.
Only You can bring new life out of deadness and sin.
Let me be like Nicodemus and seek You out
when I desperately need to make a breakthrough.
Let me lay aside all my "wisdom"
and my foolish striving in my own power.
Let me come to You honestly,
my doubts in hand, but my heart wide open
to receive the presence of Your Spirit
and the rebirth of mine.
Amen.

98 | Between the Now and the Not Yet

You are precious…in my sight, and…I love you.

ISAIAH 43:4

The great thing about real love isn't that it's blind but that it sees something more important than the outward appearance of the moment. Ask any parent. Mom looks at fourteen-year-old Chad. His table manners are a fright. His social abilities are unreliable. His room is a toxic wasteland. But in his mother's heart, Chad is a wonder in the making—a gentleman, a hero.

Dad watches his sleeping daughter. Her short legs and chubby form don't seem to belong to the worn pair of ballet slippers she keeps tucked under her bed. But Dad understands. He can already see her doing pirouettes at Carnegie Hall.

In the same way, when our heavenly Father looks at us, He sees something that's completely true about us…but may not be true *yet!* When Jesus looked at unreliable Peter, He saw a future leader of the church and nicknamed him "Rock."

In his essay "The Way of Freedom," Carlo Carretto wrote, "God loves what in us is not yet. What has still to come to birth…. And this is such a fine thing to do that God invites us to do the same. The charity which God transmits to us is this very ability to love things in a person which do not yet exist."

When you look in the mirror today, don't be deceived by what you see. God loves what is completely true about you. He loves what in you is not yet…and helps it come to be!

Food for Thought
Love sees what isn't…and helps it come to be.

A Prayer for Power

Dear God,
thank You for Your eyes, which see the best in me:
the potential in my future,
not the mistakes of my past or present.
These days we are fond of saying to one another,
"I believe in you."
But You say that to me every day,
and You really mean it!
You are not limited by time,
and You already see the me that I will become someday.
You see beyond the flaws and failures,
and You tell me they are merely proof of what wonderful changes
can and will take place in me by Your power.
Thank You, God, for loving the core of me,
the whole of me that is not yet.
Love into being
everything You want me to be.
Amen.

99 | God-Sized Prayers

Jabez was more honorable than his brothers. His mother had named him Jabez,
saying, "I gave birth to him in pain." Jabez cried out to the God of Israel, "Oh
that you would bless me and enlarge my territory! Let your hand be with me,
and keep me...from pain." And God granted his request.

1 CHRONICLES 4:9-10

Meet Jabez, one of the Bible's least-known heroes. He comes out of nowhere in the middle of the genealogies in 1 Chronicles, and in the space of two verses he does something that puts his name in God's history book. He began his life with a name that was synonymous with pain, but he ended his life getting everything he asked of God.

If you feel you've started your day—and maybe your whole life—with a whopping deficit, Jabez can be an inspiration. Despite his liabilities, or perhaps because of them, he approached his prayer life with a big dose of desperation and a great faith in God's power and goodness.

Dr. Bruce Wilkinson, a well-known Bible teacher, often advises people to pray the prayer of Jabez every day for thirty days...just to see what God will do. Why don't you ask for the world from God today?

- *O Lord, please bless me!* (a plea for God's best)
- *O Lord, please enlarge my territory!* (a plea for greater ministry and influence for God)
- *O Lord, let your hand be with me!* (a plea for God's presence and power to accomplish what would otherwise be impossible)
- *O Lord, keep me from pain!* (a plea for protection from evil and temptation and the pain they bring)

Food for Thought
Pray big prayers (you're talking to a *big* God)!

208

A PRAYER FOR POWER

Dear God,
sometimes the name "pain"
seems a fitting one for my life too.
But You are a redeemer of all who cry out to You
in pain or distress.
You reward those who start small
and are disadvantaged
but expect miracles nonetheless.
Because of who You are,
I want to be one of those who think in big terms,
who ask for the impossible.
Make me bold enough to beg You to bless me, Lord!
Give me pure motives as I reach out to receive Your blessings.
Grant me the kind of courage Jabez had.
And let my life be one that honors You
because I'm convinced of how great,
how very big,
and how very gracious You are.
Amen.

100 | O Come Let Us Adore Him!

Let everything that has breath praise the LORD.

PSALM 150:6

You've probably seen the cartoon of two women doing a power lunch. The talkative one is winding up. "Enough about me," she says to her captive audience, making a sweeping gesture in the air with her cigarette. "Tell me, what do *you* think about my new dress?"

So many of us pray like that. When we think we're finally done with our self-obsessing, we turn to thanks. But even our thanks is sometimes entirely self-centered: We thank God for all He has done *for us!*

That's where praise and worship come in. The book of Psalms is like a diary of a spiritual journey—pain, loneliness, joy, thankfulness, doubt, faith. But it culminates in a litany of one word: praise. Praise has nothing to do with how we're feeling or what's happening in our lives or what we want to ask for. It has everything and only to do with someone else: God. Finally we are focused completely on Him.

God wants us to be close to Him, to seek Him passionately. But our highest goal isn't to get what we want or even to become what we want but to respond completely and purely to God. John Piper writes in *Desiring God,* "God is most glorified in us when we are most satisfied in him." We were created to find our ultimate pleasure in our Creator, not in reaching our goals.

Today let praise and worship release God's nature and power to carry you to a higher plane of living. It's a destination that only a fortunate few experience. What a worthy destination for you, spiritual pilgrim.

A Prayer for Power

Dear God,
how wonderful it is to know You intimately,
the One and Only True God!
Forgive me when I forget Your awesomeness
because I focus so much on my neediness.
Forgive me when I fail to worship and adore all that You are
because I am busy bemoaning all that I am not.
Thank You that as I turn my eyes on You,
I glimpse the only flawless beauty and perfection in the universe.
And miraculously, as I turn my heart to worship You alone,
I somehow stumble into indescribable joy.
Grow in me this willingness, God,
to readily exchange all my self-obsession
for delighting in You.
In the days and months to come,
even as I strive to become all You created me to be,
transform me most through my self-abandoned praise of You.
May I continually join the chorus in heaven
that never stops worshiping Your name day and night, saying,
"Holy, holy, holy
is the Lord God Almighty,
who was, and is,
and is to come" (Rev. 4:8)!
Amen.

TOPICAL INDEX